PECULIAR ASPECTS OF RHINOSINUSITIS

Edited by **Gian Luigi Marseglia**
and **Davide Paolo Caimmi**

Peculiar Aspects of Rhinosinusitis
Edited by Gian Luigi Marseglia and Davide Paolo Caimmi

Published by InTech
Janeza Trdine 9, 51000 Rijeka, Croatia

Publishing Process Manager Martina Blecic

Technical Editor Teodora Smiljanic

Cover Designer InTech Design Team

Additional hard copies can be obtained from orders@intechopen.com

Peculiar Aspects of Rhinosinusitis, Edited by Gian Luigi Marseglia
and Davide Paolo Caimmi
p. cm.
ISBN 978-953-307-763-5

For EU product safety concerns:
IN TECH d.o.o., Prolaz Marije Krucifikse Kozulić 3, 51000 Rijeka, Croatia,
info@intechopen.com or visit our website at intechopen.com.

Meet the editors

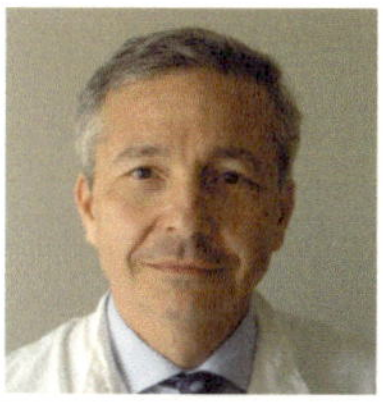

Professor Gian Luigi Marseglia was born on April 29th 1955 in Italy. He went to High School in Italy and graduated in classical studies. He finished Medical School in Italy, at the University of Pavia and he then specialized in Pediatrics, Allergy, Respiratory Physiokynesitherapy, and Infectious Diseases. He worked at the University of Lyone (France) and at the University of Brescia (Italy). Since 1991 he works at the University of Pavia, where he is a full-time Professor of Pediatrics and Head of the Department of Pediatrics and of the Allergy-Immunology Pediatric Unit. Since 2009 he is the chief of the Pediatric Program at the University of Pavia as well. He has published almost 150 articles in international journals, focusing mainly on pediatrics, allergies, respiratory and ORL diseases.

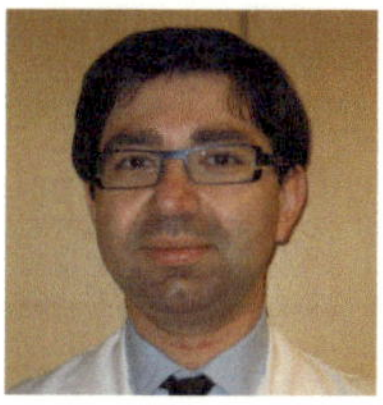

Dr. Davide Paolo Caimmi was born on April 22nd 1982 in Italy. He went to High school in Louisville (KY), United States of America, for a year, but he graduated in Italy, in classical studies. He finished Medical School in Italy, at the University of Pavia and studied for one year at the Free University of Bruxelles (Belgium). He completed his Internship and Residency in Pediatrics, at the University of Pavia (Italy), where he still works, collaborating at the same time with the Allergy Department of the University of Montpellier (France). His publications mainly concern allergies and pediatric otolaryngoiatric diseases.

Contents

Preface

Rhinitis, rhinosinusitis and respiratory diseases are among those diseases that most often lead a patient to consult a general practitioner. Unfortunately, these diseases are not always easy to manage and cure. Therefore, sometimes it becomes necessary to see a specialist. Among these three entities, rhinosinusitis is probably the one that most often creates confusion over how it should be treated and by what specialist should be evaluated.

For a long time it has been acknowledged that most of the times the disease has an infectious component, as well as the fact that is more frequent in atopic and allergic patients. Rhinosinusitis is today easily assessed by nasal endoscopy and/or sinusal computed tomography.

The management of such a condition consists of different approaches and it also depends on whether the doctor who treats the patient had a medical rather than a surgical training.

Ultimately, it has to be recalled that rhinosinusitis is an important and common disease that, among other symptoms, causes pain not only in adults but also in pediatric patients.

The clinical presentation of rhinosinusitis is heterogeneous and includes different signs and symptoms: anterior and posterior rhinorrhea, nasal obstruction, fever, halitosis, headache, facial pain, orbital pain, facial edema, edema, more or less marked in the periorbital region, cough. These symptoms, however, vary mostly on the basis of the age of the subject and of the sinuses involved in the inflammatory/infectious process.

Another aspect of the disease that needs to be taken into account when dealing with a patient presenting with rhinosinusitis is the duration of the symptoms. Considering such a feature, three forms of rhinosinusitis may be described. The acute forms are those that last less than 30 days (distinguished into mild and severe); subacute forms are those whose symptoms persist more than 30 days but less than 3 months; at last, chronic forms are those in which symptoms persist for more than 3 months. In those patients who present with chronic forms of rhinosinusitis, even though most of the times the disease is initially related to an upper respiratory tract infection, clinicians should look for an underlying diseases or an underlying condition possibly predisposing a local or systemic continuous obstruction of the hosts of the sinuses. Similarly, in those patients presenting with a persistent/recurrent rhinosinusitis or with pan-sinusitis, possible local conditions favoring the disease need to be excluded, such as a marked adenoid hypertrophy, anatomical abnormalities of the bones of the nasal cavity, nasal polyps, allergies, cystic fibrosis, immune deficiencies or ciliary dyskinesia.

At last, clinicians should be aware of the rhino-bronchial syndrome and of the need to exclude an association between sinusitis and bronchial hyper-reactivity. Most of the times, this association if discovered when a patient presenting with asthma shows a poor asthma control even after appropriate treatment. These patients show a great benefit after sinusitis treatment. Therefore, whenever such a comorbidity is found, an appropriate nasal treatment should be started.

The present monograph will therefore highlight certain specific topics concerning rhinosinusitis that usually are not clarified in other textbooks. First of all, it has to be clear that patients presenting with rhinosinusitis surely experience a worsening in their quality of life. In the first section of the book one chapter will focus on the microbiological aspects of rhinosinusitis, while two other chapters will explain the peculiar aspects of chronic rhinosinusitis and of recurrent chronic rhinosinusitis. In the second section, a chapter is dedicated to the imaging techniques to visualize the nasal sinuses and the other chapter to a medical topical type of treatment.

Rhinosinusitis is a disease that all clinicians should be aware of. The present book has the peculiarity to focus on certain aspects of the disease that are often neglected elsewhere.

Prof. Gian Luigi Marseglia
Head of the Department of Pediatrics
Head of the Allergy Immunology Pediatric Unit
University of Pavia
Foundation IRCCS Policlinico San Matteo - Pavia
Italy

Dr. Davide Caimmi
Department of Pediatrics
University of Pavia
Foundation IRCCS Policlinico San Matteo - Pavia
Italy

Part 1

Rhinosinusitis, Chronic Rhinosinusitis and Refractory Chronic Rhinosinusitis

1

Rhinosinusitis - Its Impact on Quality of Life

Petr Schalek
3rd Medical faculty of Charles University, Prague
Czech Republic

1. Introduction

Chronic rhinosinusitis (CRS) is one of the most common chronic diseases, affecting about 15% of the western population. This disease is connected with a significant health care burden having direct annual costs of about 5.8 billion dollars (Anand, 2004). These direct costs do not cover other important expenses to the individual, the community and society, such as lost time from work and / or school and the associated decreased productivity (Benninger, 2010).

CRS is an inflammatory process involving the sinonasal mucosa and defined as the presence of two or more symptoms one of which should be either nasal blockage/obstruction/congestion or nasal discharge (anterior or posterior) with

± facial pain (pressure)

± reduced smell

for more than 12 weeks, together with pathologic endoscopic findings in the middle nasal meatus (Figure 1) and/or CT changes within the ostiomeatal complex and/or sinuses (Fokkens et al., 2007). Nasal polyposis is considered a subgroup of CRS (Figure 2).

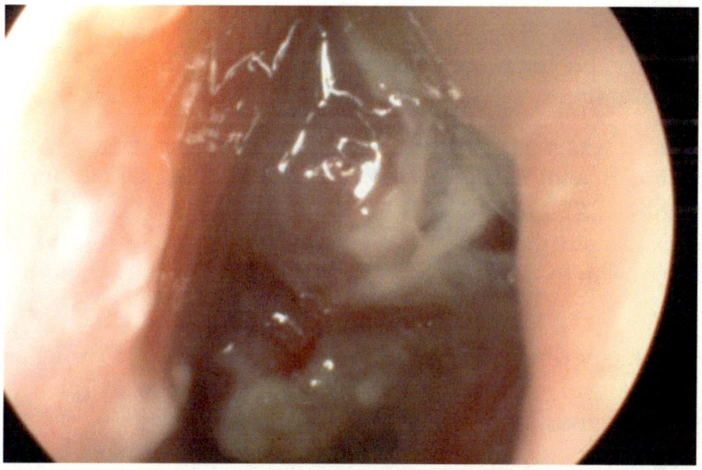

Fig. 1. Endoscopic view of chronic rhinosinusitis- edema and purulent secretion in the middle nasal meatus

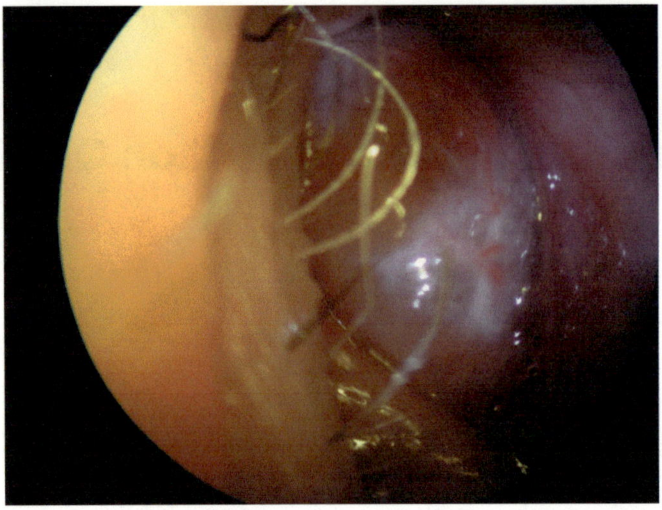

Fig. 2. Endoscopic view of nasal polyposis

Quality of life (QoL) is a unique personal experience that reflects not only health status but other factors in a patient's life which can only be described by each individual patient (Piccirillo, 2002). Quality of life may also be defined as the difference between expectations and experience (Calman, 1984). A part of the overall quality of life is health related quality of life (HRQoL), which is influenced by the health of patients and can be changed through treatment. Health related QoL may also be defined as those aspects of an individual's subjective experience that relate both directly and indirectly to health, disease, disability and impairment (Carr et al., 2001). The HRQoL is influenced by the patient's age, culture, expectations and physical and mental capabilities.

It has been shown that CRS has a significant impact on quality of life (Hopkins et al., 2009). Although the symptoms of rhinosinusitis are not life threatening they are associated with a dramatic reduction in QoL (van Oene, et al., 2007). Comparisons with other common chronic diseases revealed significantly lower scores for bodily pain and social functioning in patients with CRS compared to patients with congestive heart failure, angina, chronic obstructive pulmonary disease or back pain (Gliklich & Metson, 1995a).

When disease severity was measured using imaging and the endoscopic grading system, it was found that patients with nasal polyps (NP) appeared to have a more serious medical condition compared to CRS patients without polyps (Bhattacharyya, 2005); however, when measured using QoL instruments, and except for symptoms related to nasal congestion, patients with polyps seem to have a lighter disease burden than those without polyps (Soler & Smith, 2010).

Although there are many diagnostic methods currently available for evaluating sinonasal disease, it can not be said that the results clearly correlate with quality of life, as it is perceived by patients (Lund, 2001).

The way chronic rhinosinusitis affects daily life, from the patient's point of view, is far more important than the results of CT scans or the presence of a small polyp in an ethmoid cell (Schalek et al., 2010).

2. Instruments for quality of life assessment

The last two decades have been characterized by increasing interest in assessing the quality of life, which is related to the systematic development and validation of QoL questionnaires. Tools used to evaluate the quality of life are either generic health instruments for assessing general conditions or disease-specific questionnaires focused on symptoms of a disease.

Creation of a questionnaire is a relatively complex process involving several steps, each of which can significantly affect the final quality of the questionnaire.

The basic criteria which must be met by the questionnaire are: (i) reliability, (ii) validity, (iii) responsiveness and (iv) ease of use or feasibility.

Confirming that a particular instrument meets those criteria is a process called validation of the questionnaire. Validation studies must be performed on patients who have the same characteristics as the target population and there must be enough patients included in the validation study to make it statistically relevant.

Reliability

Reliability concerns the extent to which the questionnaire is free of random or systematic error.

Internal reliability (consistency) reflects the way individual items relate to each other. This property is determined by calculating Cronbach's α (range 0 – 1). If scale has an alpha of at least 0.7 it is considered to be reliable for group level comparisons and a value of 0.9 or more means it is suitable for assessment at the individual level (Bland & Altman, 1997).

Test-retest reliability (reproducibility) reflects stability over time with repeated testing. Questionnaires with good reproducibility should give similar results under similar conditions. This property of the questionnaire may be tested using the t- test and a Pearson or Spearman correlation coefficient or the intra-class correlation coefficient.

Validity

The questionnaire can be called valid when it measures what it is supposed to measure. Different levels of validity are distinguished.

Construct validity means that the instrument behaves according to an underlying hypothesis, i.e. the measured variables behave in a consistent way relative to theoretical and clinical expectations.

Convergent validity reflects the degree of correlation with other instruments of the same concept.

Discriminant validity reflects the ability of the questionnaire to distinguish between disease-affected groups of patients and those who are disease free.

Content validity is appropriateness and redundancy of items and scales of the instrument.

Responsiveness

Responsiveness is the sensitivity to change over time, i.e. the ability of the questionnaire to detect a change when it occurs. There are many responsiveness statistics, often it is measured by a standardized response mean- SRM (> 0.8 - high sensitivity to change).

Feasibility

Feasibility depends on a patient's understanding and willingness to complete the questionnaire. Complex, time-consuming questionnaires are usually not well received by patients, which will affect the meaningfulness of results. The feasibility can be assessed by pretesting with real patients in order to get feedback.

2.1 General health instruments

General (generic) health instruments are applicable in different diseases that can be compared regarding their impact on QoL. The following overview includes only a few of the most commonly used questionnaires, which are also frequently used to assess QoL in patients with CRS.

Short form 36 health survey (SF-36)

This questionnaire is one of the most widely used general QoL instruments. It consists of 36 items forming 8 scales (Ware & Sherbourne, 1992). The scales are: physical function, role physical, bodily pain, general health, vitality, social function, role emotional, and mental health.

Short form 12 health instrument (SF-12)

This is a shortened version of the SF-36 that contains questions from all eight SF-36 scales. Two summary scales are constructed: (i) physical and (ii) mental summary scores.

Glasgow benefit inventory (GBI)

This questionnaire was developed in 1996 (Robinson et al., 1996) and is designed to measure outcomes of surgical procedures in the field of otorhinolaryngology. The questionnaire consists of 18 items assessing the quality of life. Patients evaluate each item using the 5-grade scale: extremely positive, positive, no change, negative, extremely negative. GBI overall score the ranges from −100 to +100. Positive values indicate improvement, 0 no change of the state and negative values indicate deterioration of QoL.

2.2 Disease-specific questionnaires

This type of tool is frequently used to assess QoL in patients with CRS. Compared with general instruments they are able to capture symptoms in greater detail and are more sensitive in detecting changes after therapeutic intervention (Hopkins et al., 2009). The most frequently used validated questionnaires are listed below and their properties are summarized in Table 1.

Nasal symptom questionnaire (also Fairley nasal symptom score)

This instrument was the first (1993) validated QoL questionnaire for patients with sinonasal disease. The questionnaire consists of 12 items rated on a four-point scale (0-3). A validation study was performed on 411 patients with very good results for reliability and validity (Fairley et al., 1993). This questionnaire is not widely used, possibly due to a paucity of general health correlations.

Instrument	Developed	Language	Items	Scale	MS of CRS	Reliability	Validity	Responsi-veness	Completion (min)
Fairley NSS	1993	English	12	0-3	yes	yes	yes	yes	5
RSOM-31	1995	English	31	1-5,VAS	yes	yes	yes	yes	20
SNOT-20	2002	English, German, Japan	20	0-5	no	yes	yes	yes	7
SNOT-16	1999	English	16	0-5	no	yes	yes	yes	5
SNOT-22	2003	English, Swedish, Chnese, Czech, Danish	22	0-5	yes	yes	yes	yes	7
RSDI	1997	English, Turkish	30	0-5	yes	yes	No data	No data	5
CSS	1995	English, Chinese, Norwegian	6	0-100	no	yes	yes	yes	5
RhinoQoL	2005	English, French	17	1-5	no	yes	yes	yes	7
RSI	2003	English	20	0-5	yes	No data	yes	yes	5

Table 1. Properties of disease-specific QoL questionnaires (MS of CRS-major symptoms of CRS)

Rhinosinusitis Outcome Measure (RSOM-31), Sinonasal Outcome Test-16 (SNOT-16), SNOT-20 and SNOT-22

The RSOM-31 was developed by Piccirillo, in 1995, and contains 31 disease-specific and general items. A condensed version of this questionnaire is the SNOT-20 which has also been validated (Piccirillo et al., 2002). This questionnaire contains 20 questions, which can be divided into five subgroups (nasal symptoms, paranasal symptoms, sleep-related symptoms, and social and emotional impairment). Patients rate individual items on a six-point scale (0 - no problem, 5 - most serious problem) and in addition, they can mark which of the five items they consider to be the most important. SNOT-20 is one of the most frequently used tools and is particularly popular for its high patient compliance.

Addition questions, regarding nasal obstruction and disorders of smell, were added to SNOT-20 to produce the SNOT-22 (Figure 3). The added questions are very significant because problems with olfaction and nasal obstruction are directly related to the quality of life of patients with CRS and therapeutic interventions are designed to positively influence these two annoying symptoms. The Royal College of Surgeons of England used SNOT-22 in a National Comparative Audit of Surgery for nasal polyposis and chronic rhinosinusitis. Data for this study came from 3128 patients using questionnaire SNOT-22; the questionnaire was found easy to use and provided good discriminant validity (Hopkins et al., 2006). In 2009 the SNOT-22 was validated and recommended for routine clinical practice (Hopkins et al., 2009).

Also a 16-item version of the SNOT questionnaire has been validated. This version proved to have excellent discriminant and construct-related validity, but it does not cover all major CRS symptoms and has not gain general acceptance.

Sino-nasal outcome test-22 questionnaire

Name: **Date:**

Below you will find a list of symptoms and social/emotional consequences of your nasal disorder. We would like to know more about these problems and would appreciate you answering the following question to the best of your ability. There are no right or wrong answers, and only you can provide us with this information. Please rate your problems, as they have been over the past two weeks. Thank you for your participation.

A: Considering how severe the problem is when you experience it and how frequently it happens, please rate each item below on how 'bad' it is by circling the number that corresponds with how you feel using this scale ➔	**No problem**	**Very mild problem**	**Mild or slight problem**	**Moderate problem**	**Severe problem**	**Problem as bad as it can be**
1. Need to blow nose	0	1	2	3	4	5
2. Sneezing	0	1	2	3	4	5
3. Runny nose	0	1	2	3	4	5
4. Cough	0	1	2	3	4	5
5. Post nasal discharge (dripping at the back of your nose)	0	1	2	3	4	5
6. Thick nasal discharge	0	1	2	3	4	5
7. Ear fullness	0	1	2	3	4	5
8. Dizziness	0	1	2	3	4	5
9. Ear pain	0	1	2	3	4	5
10. Facial pain/pressure	0	1	2	3	4	5
11. Difficulty falling asleep	0	1	2	3	4	5
12. Waking up at night	0	1	2	3	4	5
13. Lack of a good night's sleep	0	1	2	3	4	5
14. Waking up tired	0	1	2	3	4	5
15. Fatigue	0	1	2	3	4	5
16. Reduced productivity	0	1	2	3	4	5
17. Reduced concentration	0	1	2	3	4	5
18. Frustrated/restless/ irritable	0	1	2	3	4	5
19. Sad	0	1	2	3	4	5
20. Embarrassed	0	1	2	3	4	5
21. Sense of taste/smell	0	1	2	3	4	5
22. Blockage/congestion of nose	0	1	2	3	4	5

Fig. 3. The SNOT-22 questionnaire

Chronic sinusitis survey (CSS)

One of the most frequently used instruments was developed by Gliklich and Metson in 1995 (Gliklich & Metson, 1995b). The CSS consists of two parts, symptom-based and medication-based (Figure 4). When using the CSS, patients do not assess the severity of symptoms, but their duration, which, together with a limited number of questions can be regarded as a disadvantage (Morley & Sharp, 2006). Furthermore the questionnaire does not include any questions related to olfaction.

Chronic Sinusitis Survey-CSS

1. During the past 8 weeks, how many weeks have you had:
   a. Sinus headaches, facial pain or pressure
   0 weeks 1-2 weeks 3-4 weeks 7-8 weeks
   b. Nasal drainage or postnasal drip
   0 weeks 1-2 weeks 3-4 weeks 7-8 weeks
   c. Nasal congestion or difficulty breathing through the your nose
   0 weeks 1-2 weeks 3-4 weeks 7-8 weeks
2. During the past 8 weeks, how many weeks have you taken
   a. Antibiotics
   0 weeks 1-2 weeks 3-4 weeks 7-8 weeks
   b. Nasal sprays prescribed by your doctor
   0 weeks 1-2 weeks 3-4 weeks 7-8 weeks
   c. Sinus medications in pill form (such as antihistamines,deconestants)
   0 weeks 1-2 weeks 3-4 weeks 7-8 weeks

Fig. 4. Chronic Sinusitis Survey-CSS

Rhinosinusitis disability index (RSDI)

The questionnaire (Figure 5) was developed in 1997 by Benninger and Senior (Benninger & Senior, 1997). RSDI uses three subscales (emotional, physical and functional) to combine measurements of general health status and disease-specific QoL. The questionnaire is characterized by excellent test-retest reliability, good internal consistency, good construct, discriminant and content validity.

The rhinosinusitis disability index (RSDI) domains and items

Physical

The pain or pressure in my face makes it difficult for me to concentrate
3. The pain in my eyes makes it difficult for me to read
4. I have difficulty stooping over to lift objects because of face pressure
5. Because of my problem I have difficulty with strenuous yard work and housework
6. Straining increases or worsens my problem
7. I am inconvenienced by my chronic runny nose
8. Food does not taste good because of my change in smell
9. My frequent sniffing is irritating to my friends and family
10. Because of my problem I don't sleep well
11. I have difficulty with exertion due to my nasal obstruction
12. My sexual activity is affected by my problem

Functional

Because of my problem I feel handicapped
13. Because of my problem I feel restricted in performance of my routine daily activities
14. Because of my problem I restrict my recreational activities

15. Because of my problem I feel frustrated
16. Because of my problem I feel fatigued
17. Because of my problem I avoid traveling
18. Because of my problem I miss work or social activities
19. My outlook on the world is affected by my problem
20. Because of my problem I find it difficult to focus my attention away from my problem and on other things

Emotional

Because of my problem I feel stressed in relationships with friends and family

21. Because of my problem I feel confused
22. Because of my problem I have difficulty paying attention
23. Because of my problem I avoid being around people
24. Because of my problem I am frequently angry
25. Because of my problem I do not like to socialize
26. Because of my problem I frequently feel tense
27. Because of my problem I frequently feel irritable
28. Because of my problem I am depressed
29. My problem places stress on my relationships with members of my family or friends

Fig. 5. Rhinosinusitis disability index- RSDI

Rhinosinusitis symptom inventory (RSI)

One of the more recent questionnaires (Bhattacharyya, 2005) was developed mainly to evaluate improvement of QoL after treatment. The instrument assesses major and minor symptoms of CRS on a six-point scale. Simultaneously, medication use, doctor visits and work absences (directly related to CRS) are recorded.

Rhinosinusitis quality of life survey (RhinoQoL)

This 17-item questionnaire is based on the CSS and the questioning system of both instruments is identical. The RhinoQoL does not contain questions regarding olfaction disturbances, which is one of major symptoms of CRS. The questionnaire was validated by Atlas on a population of 50 patients (Atlas et al., 2005).

There is also one important question concerning QoL measurement: How is a clinically significant change of health-related QoL defined? Statistically significant improvement does not always mean clinically relevant improvement as perceived by an individual patient. A concept called the minimal important difference helps address this problem. It is defined as the smallest change in QoL that patients perceive as beneficial, in the absence of side effects or excessive cost (Juniper at al., 1994). Prior studies measuring acute pain have shown that the minimal important difference for acute pain is between 0.9 and 1.3 on a 10-point scale. Recent studies reporting scaled symptom scores by Ling and Kountakis (Ling & Kountakis, 2007) and Bhattacharyya (Bhattacharyya, 2005) easily reach this threshold of clinical relevance. For the general health instrument SF-36, 10 to 12.5 points (100-point scale) represents the minimum change believed to be clinically relevant (Wyrwick et al., 2005).

Using statistical constructs, the minimal important difference has been defined as greater than half a standard deviation of the baseline QoL value for the given population. Recently Soler and Smith (Soler & Smith, 2010) summarized minimal important differences for disease specific QoL instruments (Table 2).

Questionnaire	Score Range	MCID
RSDI total	0-120	≥10.35
RSDI Physical	0-44	≥3.80
RSDI Functional	0-36	≥3.45
RSDI Emotionals	0-40	≥4.20
CSS total	0-100	≥9.75
CSS Symptoms	0-100	≥13.25
CSS Medications	0-100	≥12.60
SNOT-22	0-110	≥8.90

Table 2. Minimal important differences (MCID) for disease-specific QoL questionnaires (Soler & Smith, 2010)

Another important issue may be how to choose a particular tool for evaluating QoL in patients, regarding assessment of therapeutic effects or comparison of two or more therapeutic modalities on QoL.

A review of Chester and Sindwani, from 2007 (Chester & Sindwani, 2007), demonstrates that of the 18 QoL instruments used to evaluate the outcomes of endoscopic sinus surgery (ESS), only 5 were used more than twice: CSS (12 studies), SNOT-20 (11 studies), SF-36 (10 studies), RSI (4 Studies) and RSDI (3 studies).

Gill et al. proposed three recommendations to improve the measurement of quality of life: (i) use of global ratings, ideally one for general QoL and one for disease-specific QoL; (ii) severity and importance of symptoms must be rated; (iii) a possibility for patients to add other annoying symptoms (Gill & Feinstein, 1994). This recommendation takes into account the study of Morley et al, which suggests the SNOT-22 was the best tool for treatment evaluation, especially the after ESS (Morley & Sharp, 2006). This study was published in 2006, before the SNOT-22 had been validated. SNOT-22 fully corresponds to the recommendation of Gill and his co-workers - it includes questions regarding sinonasal symptoms, covers the major symptoms of CRS and also includes questions assessing the overall quality of life. It allows patients to easily assess the severity of symptoms and select the symptoms that are most important from their point of view. In addition, patients have the opportunity to present other troublesome symptoms that are not listed in the questionnaire.

The study of van Oene et al. focused on the issue of quality of disease specific QoL instruments (van Oene, 2007). Only questionnaires that clearly meet the following criteria were included in the study: (i) the questionnaire must be designed for adults with CRS and (ii) must cover all three aspects of HRQL-physical, functional and psychosocial. Parameters of the questionnaire, i.e. construction, description, feasibility, validation study and psychometric properties are all ranked using a points system. Criteria were fulfilled only for

RSOM-31, SNOT-16, SNOT-20, RSDI and RhinoQoL. The highest scores were achieved by RSOM-31 and SNOT-20. The questionnaire SNOT-22 was not enrolled because it had not yet been validated. CSS and RSDI did not meet the definition of a HRQL questionnaire. The authors point out the importance of the relationship between the characteristics of the questionnaire and the purpose for which it should be used. For example, for use in clinical practice, reliability of the instrument is essential, while for the purposes of clinical research, responsiveness (for longitudinal study) or discriminant validity (for cross-sectional studies) may be critical.

3. How the Rhinosinusitis afffects the quality of life

Symptoms of CRS can be disabling and lead to significant impairment of QoL. The most common reported symptom in CRS is nasal congestion/obstruction (Bhattacharyya, 2003). This symptom is accompanied by nasal discharge (anterior or posterior), reduction or loss of olfaction, facial pain or pressure and headaches, which were reported as the most disabling (Soler et al., 2008). These symptoms can impact all activities (work, leisure and sleep) of CRS patients. It is reasonable to expect that individual CRS symptoms can result in more complex problems such as sleep disturbances, psychological disorders (changes in mood, depression, and anxiety), fatigue, and sexual dysfunction.

3.1 Sleep disturbance and fatigue

Although sleep impairment has been studied less in CRS compared to allergic rhinitis, it is obvious that CRS is associated with this problem as well (Craig et al., 2008).

Also, a recent study by Benninger demonstrated that patients with CRS have significantly reduced sleep activity scores on the Rhinosinusitis Disability Index (Benninger et al., 2010).

In a population-based, case-control study, patients with nasal polyposis had a 2-fold higher risk of sleep disturbances than controls (Serrano et al., 2005). This is further supported by a study that approached it from the other way around; in a study of general medical outpatients, an increased prevalence of CRS symptoms in patients with unexplained chronic fatigue was observed (Chester, 2003). Thus, sleep impairment is a significant issue for CRS patients and questions regarding quality of the sleep have been incorporated in many disease-specific QoL questionnaires.

Nasal congestion/obstruction is thought to be a major cause of sleep impairment. This bothersome CRS symptom is usually worse at night, which is result of the lower position of the patient's head. Additionally, the overnight decline of serum cortisol levels can contribute to night-time nasal congestion. Nasal obstruction in healthy subjects leads to apneas and hypopneas (Suratt et al., 1986). Other CRS symptoms (e.g. discharge, facial pain and headache) can also reduce sleep quality.

It is also assumed that inflammatory mediators of CRS probably play a direct role in sleep disturbances (Craig et al., 2008).

There is a clear relationship between sleep impairment and daily fatigue. Poorly sleeping patients would be expected to experience fatigue and improved sleep should have a positive influence on fatigue.

3.2 Depression

Brandsted and Sindwani demonstrated that 25% of consecutively diagnosed CRS patients were also treated for depression, which is higher than in the general population (10 - 16%) (Brandsted & Sindwani, 2007). In this study the authors also compared the QoL of CRS patients with depression to a control group of CRS patients without depression. The results showed significantly poorer disease-specific and overall QoL scores in depressed CRS patients (both pre- and postoperatively).

Additionally, Mace reported lower preoperative and postoperative QoL scores in CRS patients with depression compared to non-depressed patients but with comparable improvements after endoscopic sinus surgery in both groups (Mace et al., 2008).

Wasan identified high levels of anxiety and depression in patients who undergo evaluation for CRS using the Rhinosinusitis Symptom Inventory and the Hospital Anxiety and Depression Scale (Wasan et al., 2007).

In conclusion depression is frequently associated with CRS and contributes to lower overall QoL in CRS patients, although it is likely that the diseases are independent (Rudmik & Smith, 2011).

3.3 Sexual dysfunction

Sexual activity is another important aspect of QoL. It is not hard to imagine that patients with nasal obstruction, discharge, reduced olfaction, facial pressure and sleep deficits would have an altered sex life compared to healthy controls. The Rhinosinusitis Disability Index (RSDI) is a disease-specific QoL questionnaire which has one question which directly addresses the impact of sinonasal disease on sexual function.

There are few studies dealing with sexual function in patients with sinonasal disease. Two trials investigating the influence of allergic rhinitis on sexual function, demonstrated lower scores for sexual function in patients suffering from allergic rhinitis compared those without sinonasal disease or with non-allergic rhinitis or anatomical obstruction. Although CRS was not specially evaluated in these studies, the results suggest that CRS may have similar negative effects on sexual function. (Benninger & Benninger, 2009; Kirmaz et al., 2005).

Benninger, using the Rhinosinusitis Disability Index, has provided data (on level of evidence IIIb) showing that functional endoscopic surgery for CRS has a positive impact on sexual function (Benninger et al., 2010).

3.4 Olfactory dysfunction

Smell disturbance is a common symptom affecting 61 - 83% of patients with CRS. Patient with olfactory impairment often report problems preparing food, decreased appetite, and a decreased sense of self-hygiene. Patients are also not able to detect spoiled foods and safety hazards such as smoke, chemicals, and gas leaks (Litvack et al., 2009). Moreover there are some professions dependent on good olfactory function (chefs, professional tasters, fireman, plumbers, etc.) and loss of smell in those occupations can be debilitating.

Although humans and other primates are regarded as primarily "optical animals" with a relatively undeveloped sense of smell, recent studies indicate that humans seem to use olfactory communication, particularly, in interpersonal relationships (Grammer et al., 2005). Perception of substances such as pheromones may modulate changes in interpersonal perception and individual mood, behavior and physiology (Havlicek et al., 2010).

4. Effect of rhinosinusitis treatment on quality of life

The effect of surgical treatment on QoL in patients with CRS has been documented fairly well (Metson & Glicklich, 1998; Salhab et al., 2004; Smith et al., 2005; Ling & Kountakis, 2007).

A review by Smith et al. assessed the effect of surgical treatment of CRS on symptoms and QoL in patients with CRS. Improvement of quality of life or symptoms was demonstrated in all 45 enrolled studies, 11 studies were prospective, and in five, a validated QoL questionnaire was used (Smith. et al., 2005).

Ling and Kountakis (Ling & Kountakis, 2007) showed a greater than 80% improvement in symptoms of CRS from baseline, when measured using a visual analogue scale, 12 months after ESS. These authors also used SNOT-22 scores that showed improvement by as much as 77%, postoperatively.

Improvement of both major and minor symptoms of CRS after ESS was also shown by Bhattacharyya (Bhattacharyya, 2005) using the RSDI (100 patients, average follow-up = 19 months).

Litvack (Litvack et al., 2007) showed that both primary and revision endoscopic surgery equally improved QoL (the RSDI and CSS questionaires were the QoL instruments used in the trial).

A prospective audit conducted on 3128 patients undergoing surgery for CRS also demonstrated a significant improvement of QoL over a 36-month follow-up (SNOT-22) (Hopkins et al., 2006).

Proimos (Proimos et al., 2010) demonstrated improvement of QoL in 86 patients with CRS with nasal polyps and asthma, 12 months after ESS. In this study SNOT-22 was used and additionally, the 5 most important items of SNOT, from the patient's point of view, were evaluated. The results confirmed that ESS satisfied expectations of patients regarding control of most of the important symptoms and a positive influenced on their overall QoL.

In a recent multi-institutional, prospective study, Smith et al. (Smith et al., 2010) demonstrated clinically significant improvement of QoL (CSS and RSDI questionnaires were used in 302 patients, mean ESS follow-up = 17.4 months). Authors of this study also tried to find predictive factors for QoL outcomes after ESS. They used a multivariate logistic regression model to examine predictors of clinically significant improvement of QoL. In this predictive model, after all co-factors were evaluated (e.g. comorbidities, demographic factors, and results of diagnostics tests), surprisingly, only primary or revision surgery was clearly predictive. The authors concluded that clinical phenotype did not provide outcome-predictive information and other factors with possible predictive importance should be investigated.

There is a relative lack of documentation regarding improvement of QoL after medical treatment of CRS. Similarly, there are insufficient data regarding comparisons of effects of different medical and surgical treatments on QoL. The lack of well-formed, prospective, randomized, controlled trials, concerning medical treatment can lead to the idea that surgical treatment of CRS has a better effect on QoL than medical treatments (Ragab et al., 2010).

Also the fact that surgical treatment should only be indicated for patients with a more severe course of disease, resistant to medical treatment, makes any comparison of effect of treatment on QoL more complicated.

A study by Lund et al. (Lund et al., 2004) showed no significant difference in the score on a disease-specific questionnaire (Chronic Sinusitis survey-CSS) in patients with CRS without NP, treated for 20 months with intranasal budesonide compared to placebo. In the same study, a significant difference between the two groups was found only in the general health subscale of SF-36 General Health Questionnaire, but no significant difference in the other subscales were observed.

Alobid et al. (Alobid et al., 2006) assessed the effect of treatment with oral and intranasal steroids on the quality of life of patients with CRS with nasal polyposis. The patients, after a short-course of oral prednisone, demonstrated a significant improvement in QoL in all domains (compared with base line and the control group) using the general-health QoL instrument SF-36. The improvement was sustained by intranasal steroids after 12, 24 and 48 months. The study was conducted on 60 patients who were compared with a control group (18 patients) without treatment.

The same group (Alobid et al., 2005) compared, in a randomized trial, medical treatment (53 patients, oral prednisone for two weeks) and surgical treatment (56 patients undergoing ESS) of CRS with nasal polyps. Both groups received intranasal budesonide for 12 months after intervention. At 6 and 12 months, a significant improvement in the QoL, measured again using the SF-36, was observed in both the medical and surgical group.

Ragab et al. in a recent prospective, randomized, controlled trial evaluated and compared the effect of medical and surgical treatment of CRS on QoL (Ragab et al., 2010). The study was conducted on ninety CRS patients with and without polyps randomized into medical and surgical groups. The medical group was treated with erythromycin (12 week course), alkaline nasal douches and intranasal steroids. In addition, 3 patients with polyps were prescribed a course of short-term oral steroids. The extent of endoscopic sinus surgery was tailored to the extent of the disease in the surgical group. Following ESS, all patients were prescribed a two-week course of erythromycin and alkaline douches and intranasal steroids as long-term therapy. Quality of life was assessed using the disease specific instrument SNOT-22 and the general health instrument SF-36 before randomization and after 6 and 12 months. A significant improvement in the SNOT score was recorded, without statistically significant difference between medical and surgical group after 6 and 12 month. Also, the SF-36 demonstrated a significant improvement in the QoL in seven out of eight domains. Only physical functioning did not change significantly from the baseline. Furthermore this study does not support the fact that polyps represent a poor prognostic factor for efficacy of treatment, as has been suggested in previous studies (Kennedy, 1992; Sobol et al., 1998).

In conclusion, the presented data provides evidence that both maximal medical and surgical therapy improve the QoL of CRS patients. CRS should be targeted with maximal medical therapy as the first step and surgery should be reserved for refractory cases.

5. The correlation between quality of life and the results of other measurements in chronic rhinosinusitis

The relationship between health-related QoL and the results of other examinations of CRS is not entirely clear. Although we might intuitively expect that patients with worse CT and endoscopic findings would have a lower quality of life, results of available studies do not confirm this fact. Also, the influence of CRS symptoms on QoL, relative to treatment, cannot be predicted from endoscopic or CT scores.

The lack of correlation between objective assessment and subjective perception of QoL is not unique to CRS, but can also be seen in such disorders as bronchial asthma, obstructive sleep apnea and low back pain (Soler & Smith 2010).

5.1 Imaging methods

Bhattacharyya et al. failed to demonstrate a correlation between CT scores and the SNOT-20 (Bhattacharyya et al., 1997) in 221 patients referred for CT scans.

Wabnitz et al. failed to demonstrate a significant correlation between CT scores based on the commonly used Lund-Mackay staging (score range 0-24) and the SNOT-20 QoL questionnaire in 221 patients indicated for CRS surgery; the study also found no correlation between the SNOT-20 and symptom scores (visual analog scale-VAS) (Wabnitz et al., 2005).

In a study by Holbrook et al., they tried to correlate the RSOM-31 questionnaire and the Lund Mackay CT scores. In this study patients were also asked to locate their sinus pain and pressure. The study was not able to demostrate a correlation between QoL scores and CT findings or between CT findings and areas of facial pain (Holbrook et al., 2005).

Hopkins et al. found a small, clinically insignificant association between Lund-Mackay scores and SNOT-22. In the study, CT findings from 1840 patients with CRS were reviewed and the results were consistent with the above mentioned studies. In this study, a small but significant association between CT scores and postoperative improvement on the SNOT-22 was found, which indicates that patients with lower preoperative CT scores benefit more from surgical treatment (Hopkins et al., 2007).

In conclusion CT scans measure a different aspect of CRS than QoL and, of itself, cannot be an indication for surgery. It is necessary for preoperative assessment of the extent of disease and identification of anatomical landmarks, but it should not be used for prediction or localization of CRS symptoms.

5.2 Rhinoendoscopy

A varying degree of correlation has been shown between improvement of sinonasal symptoms and results from endoscopic examinations after ESS (Giger et al., 2004; Wright & Agrawal, 2007).

Wright et al. showed a slight correlation between endoscopic scores based on the Lund-Kennedy and Sinus Symptom Questionnaire, 1, 3 and 6 months after ESS. However, this study did not show a significant correlation between postoperative endoscopic examination and the CSS (Wright & Agrawal, 2007). Studies evaluating the effect of non-surgical treatment also demonstrated no correlation between RSDI and endoscopic scores (Birch et al., 2001).

A recent study by Mace et al. focused on the correlation between endoscopic scores and HRQOL in patients after ESS. This study evaluated the results of endoscopic scores based on the Lund-Kennedy (score range 0 – 20) and two HRQoL questionnaires, RSDI, and CSS, in 102 patients preoperatively and 12 months after ESS. Changes in endoscopic scores were significantly correlated with improvement in RSDI total scores, physical RSDI subscale scores and functional RSDI subscale scores and CSS symptom scores. On the contrary, no correlation was observed among RSDI emotional subscale scores and CSS medication subscale scores and CSS total scores. When the groups of patients with and without nasal polyps (NP) were assessed separately, patients with CRS + NP (36 patients) demonstrated a significantly stronger correlation. In contrast, the group of patients without NP demonstrated no correlation between improved endoscopic scores and any of the HRQoL instruments. The authors concluded that the reason for the significant increase in quality of life in patients with NP was related to improvement in nasal breathing, olfaction, and relief of the facial pressure. The results of multivariate modeling used in this study revealed that the amount of improvement on the HRQoL can be explained by relatively small improvements on the endoscopic score. For example, with a single point improvement in the endoscopic score, RSDI total scores would be expected to improve by 1.03 units (Mace et al., 2010).

In conclusion the improvement on HRQoL is a complex process that cannot be explained only by improved endoscopic findings.

5.3 Histopathologic findings

The studies in this issue are focused primarily on the correlation between eosinophilic inflammation of the paranasal sinus mucosa and other parameters indicative of disease severity (particularly CT scan, endoscopy, examination of olfaction). The presence of eosinophilic inflammation, defines a subgroup of CRS, which is refractory to conservative and surgical treatment and knowledge of the eosinophilic status can provide information regarding the severity of the disease and help in choosing an appropriate treatment strategy.

Studies by Kountakis and Baudoin failed to demonstrate a correlation between the eosinophil count and the severity of CRS symptoms (Kountakis et al., 2004; Baudoin et al., 2006).

Soler et al. showed mucosal eosinophilia correlated with disease severity expressed by CT, endoscopy and Smell Identification Test (SIT). In contrast to this finding, they did not demonstrate a correlation between eosinophilia and two disease-specific QoL questionnaires (RSDI, CSS) or with the general QoL instrument, Short Form Health Survey, SF-36. Moreover, the study showed no correlation between QoL and any other cell, stromal and epithelial marker of inflammation (Soler et al., 2009).

Another study by Soler et al. focused on the comparison of quality of life in patients with and without eosinophilia after ESS. In accordance with the previous study, no baseline differences were observed for any QoL Instrument (RSDI, CSS, SF-36) between patients with and without eosinophilia. Although both groups showed improved quality of life after surgery, a clear trend towards less improvement in patients with eosinophilia was observed (Soler et al., 2010).

A recent study by Hai (Hai et al., 2010) indicated that patients with biofilm CRS significantly improved their QoL after ESS, however the degree of biofilm reduction did not correlate with QoL.

From the above, the QoL measurement, in the context of histopathological findings, again shows some differences between other parameters, which are often used as indicators of disease severity.

5.4 Olfactory function

It is generally considered that the loss of smell, a typical CRS symptom, significantly contributes to reduced quality of life (Deems et al., 1991; Temmel et al., 2002; Miwa et al., 2001; Bramerson et al., 2007). From this perspective, the work of Litvack et al., which deals with correlations of olfaction disturbances with other parameters of CRS severity, is interesting. Not surprisingly, endoscopic and CT scores correlated moderately with olfactory scores. In contrast, however, there was no correlation between olfactory function and disease-specific (RSDI, CSS) QoL questionnaires or the general health-related (SF-36) QoL questionnaire (Litvack et al., 2009). In this particular study the reason for these results may be the relatively limited ability of the selected questionnaires to assess olfactory function. Neither the CSS nor the SF-36 contains any questions regarding olfaction, and only one question on the RSDI addresses this issue. A similar deficiency can be found in other CRS-specific validated instruments including the RSOM and SNOT-20.

5.5 Mucociliary transport

It can be assumed that improved mucociliary transport should positively affect the symptoms of CRS. Boatsman et al. conducted a study that examined the correlation between the results of SNOT-20 and the saccharine test of mucociliary transport. In this study no significant correlation between the parameters was demonstrated. Moreover, no correlation between the individual domain scores and mucociliary clearance time was shown (Boatsman et al. 2006).

Similar research by Naxakis, also failed to demonstrate a correlation between mucociliary velocity, and QoL (SNOT-20) in patients after surgical and conservative treatment of CRS (Naxakis et al., 2009).

Clinicians are used to basing their diagnostic and therapeutic decisions on the results of objective tests, particularly CT and endoscopic findings while letting patient specific symptoms slip into the background. It is important to realize, however, that it is the symptoms that force patients to seek medical care and it is the symptoms of CRS that significantly influence and reduce their quality of life. The above listed data clearly shows that quality of life is a unique, multidimensional tool that can be used to assess the severity of the disease. The relationship between QoL measured results and results of other "objective" investigations clearly supports the fact that QoL evaluation measures different aspects of the disease.

6. Barriers and limitations of the quality of life measurement

Despite the undeniable benefit of evaluating the quality of life in diagnosis and treatment of CRS, there are some opposition regarding the routine use of this tool in clinical practice. Specific objections include:

Measurement of QoL takes too much time

Completing the most frequently used questionnaire takes less than 10 minutes. When the patient takes the questionnaire for the first time, it is necessary to educate them; therefore, the first measurement may take a little longer. The time devoted to patient instruction will be appreciated during repeated examinations, which are usually less time consuming. Inclusion of QoL measurements in routine practice is also a function of organization; it is time-effective, for example, to ask patients to fill out the questionnaire while they are waiting to be seen.

Examination of quality of life is too subjective and therefore unreliable

Outcomes rated by a clinician may be thought to be more reliable than measures rated by a patient. However, we should realize that grading of the symptoms by a clinician is prone to error. A study comparing the severity of a disease from the patient's viewpoint vs. a doctor's viewpoint, demonstrated that patients evaluate their condition as being more serious (Scadding & Wiliams, 2008); 124 patients with allergic rhinitis participated in the study; however, it can be assumed that similar results would be observed in patients with CRS as well.

We should always keep in mind that it is the symptoms that reduce the quality of life for the patient, and it is the symptoms that motivate the patient to see the doctor; no one else other than the patients, is more competent to comment on how they perceive their symptoms and how the symptoms impact their life.

The results of QoL measurements do not correlate with outcomes of objective tests

As already mentioned the evaluation of quality of life evaluates a different aspect of the disease. Symptoms and QoL are the result of interactions between many factors, of which, measurable biological and physiological variables are only a part (Figure 6) (Wilson & Clearly, 1995). For these same reasons, measurement of QoL cannot serve as a predictor of treatment outcomes.

Limitations of QoL measurements

It should be emphasized that QoL measurement is only a part of the rhinology examination and cannot substitute for other tests. For instance, a preoperative CT scan is always necessary, as well as imaging in cases of impending complication from sinusitis, which may endanger the patient's life while causing relatively minor subjective complaints. Surgery to improve nasal patency should be always associated with an objective parameter (rhinomanometry, inspiratory peak flow) and so on.

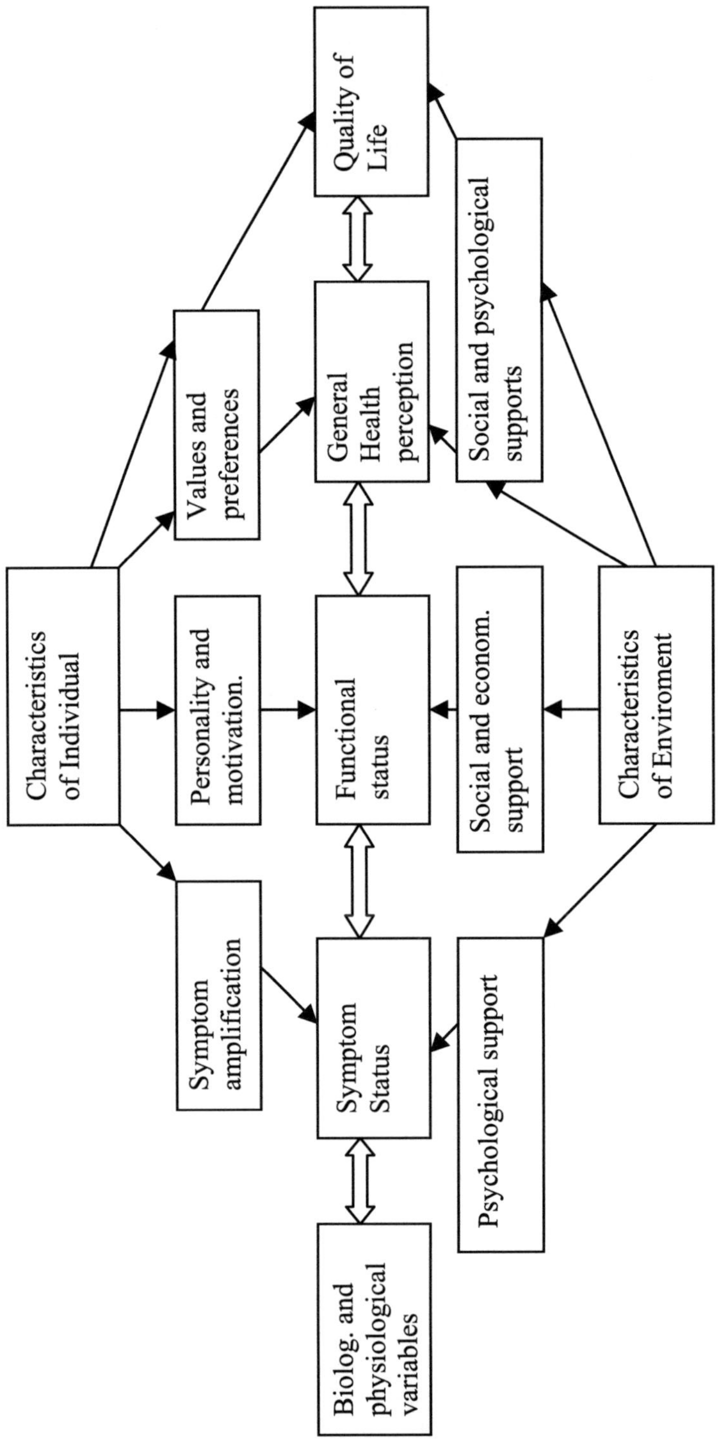

Fig. 6. Interactions between factors influencing quality of life (Wilson & Clearly, 1995)

7. Conclusion

CRS is a disease with a high incidence, which significantly affects the quality of life. Quality of life of patients is negatively influenced not only by CRS symptoms (nasal congestion, discharge, facial pain and pressure, headache, anosmia), but it is also accompanied by elevated rates of depression, anxiety, sexual and sleep disturbances and fatigue. The primary interest of treatment of rhinologic diseases is to improve the quality of life of patients.

In the last two decades there has been a significant increase in interest in measuring quality of life using specially developed, validated questionnaires. These tools allow the patient to express how CSR affects their daily life. In addition, by measuring the quality of life, we can evaluate the effect of treatment or compare different treatment methods.

Quality of life is the result of interactions among many factors and "measurable" biological and physiological factors are only part of the QoL equation. It is therefore not surprising that the quality of life does not always correlate with results of other tests that we perform on CRS patients.

The available data shows that both conservative and surgical treatments lead to improvement in the quality of life.

We can conclude by saying that measurement of quality of life should become a routine part of our everyday practice and the results should be considered in context with other indicators of disease severity. Moreover, in some countries, the data obtained by measuring the quality of life of CRS patients may be compulsory for use in evaluating treatment effectiveness and can thus influence payments to medical care providers.

8. Abbreviations

CRS	Chronic Rhinosinusitis
CSS	Chronic Sinusitis Survey
ESS	Endoscopic Sinus Surgery
GBI	Glasgow Benefit Inventory
HRQoL	Health-related Quality of Life
NP	Nasal Polyposis
QoL	Quality of Life
RhinoQoL	Rhinosinusitis Quality of Life Survey
RSOM	Rhinosinusitis Outcome Measures
RSDI	Rhinosinusitis Disability Index
RSI	Rhinosinusitis Symptom Inventory
SF-12	Short Form 12 Health Instrument
SF-36	Short Form 36 Health Survey
SNOT	Sinonasal Outcome Test
SRM	Standardized Response Mean

9. References

Alobid, I., Benitez, P., Bernal-Sperkelsen, M. et al. (2005). Nasal polyposis and its impact on quality of life: comparison between the effects of medical and surgical treatments. *Allergy*, Vol. 60:452-458.

Alobid, I., Benitez, P., Pujols, L. et al. (2006). Severe nasal polyposis and its impact on quality of life. The effect of short course of oral steroid followed by long-term intranasal steroids tretment. *Rhinology*, Vol. 44:8-13.

Anand, VK. (2004). Epidemiology and economic impact of rhinosinusitis. *Ann Otol Rhinol Laryngol*, Suppl, 193:3-5.

Atlas, SJ., Metson, RB, Singer, DE. et al. (2005). Validity of a new health-related quality of life instrument for patients with chronic rhinosinusitis. *Laryngoscope*, Vol. 115:846-854.

Baudoin, T., Cupic, H., Geber, G., et al. (2006). Histopathlogic parameters as predictors of response to endoscopic sinus surgery in nonallergic patients with chronic rhinosinusitis. *Otolaryngol Head Neck Surg*, Vol. 134:761-766.

Benninger, MS.& Senior, BA. (1997). The development of Rhinosinusitis Disability Index. *Arch Otolaryngol Head Neck Surg*, Vol.123:1175-1179.

Benninger, MS & Benninger, RM. (2009). The impact of allergic rhinitis on sexual activity, sleep and fatigue. *Allergy Asthma Proc*, Vol. 30:358-365.

Benninger, MS, Khalid, AN, Benninger, RM et al. (2010). Surgery for chronic rhinosinusitis may improve sleep and sexual function. *Laryngoscope*, Vol. 120:1696-1700.

Bhattacharyya, N., Piccirillo, J. & Wippold, FJ. (1997). Relationship between patient-based descriptions od sinusitis and paranasal sinus CT. *Arch Otolaryngol Head Neck Surg*, Vol. 123:1189-1192.

Bhattacharyya, N. (2003). The economic burden and symptom manifestations of chronic rhinosinusitis. *Am J Rhinol*, Vol. 17:27-32.

Bhattacharyya, N. (2005). Symptom outcomes after endoscopic sinus surgery for chronic rhinosinusitis. *Arch Otolaryngol Head Neck Surg*, Vol. 130:329-334.

Birch, DS, Saleh, HA, Wodehouse, T. et al. (2001). Assesing the quality of life for patients with chronic rhinosinusitis using the "Rhinosinusitis Disability Index". *Rhinology*, Vol. 39:191-196.

Bland, JM. & Altman, DG. (1997). Cronbach's alpha. BMJ, Vol. 314:572.

Boatsman, JE., Calhoun, KH. & Ryan, MW. (2006). Relationship between rhinosinusitis symptoms and mucociliary transport. *Otolaryngol Head Neck Surg*, Vol.134:491-493.

Bramerson, A., Nordin, S. & Bende, M. (2007). Clinical experience with patients wizh olfactory complaints, and their quality of life. *Acta Oto-Laryngologica* , Vol. 127:167-174.

Brandsted, R. & Sindwani, R. (2007). Impact of depression on disease-specific symptoms and quality of life in patients with chronic rhinosinusitis. *Am J Rhinol*, Vol. 21:50-54.

Calman, KC. (1984). Quality of life in cancer patients- an hypothesis. *J Med Ethics*, Vol. 10:124-127.

Carr, AJ., Gibson, BA. & Robinson, PG. (2001). Is quality of life determined by expectations or experience? *BMJ*, Vol. 322:1240-1243.

Chester, AC. (2003). Symptoms of rhinosinusitis in patients with unexplained chronic fatigue or bodily pain: a pilot study. *Arch Inter Med*, Vol. 163:1832-1836.

Chester, AC. & Sindwani, R. (2007). Symptom outcome in Endoscopic sinus surgery: A systematic review of measurements methods. Laryngoscope, Vol. 117:2239-2243.

Craig, TJ., Ferguson, BJ. & Krouse, JH. (2008). Sleep impairment in allergic rhinitis, rhinosinusitis and nasal polyposis. *American Journal of Otolaryyngology-Head and Neck Medicine and Surgery*, Vol. 29:209-217.

Deems, DA, Doty, RL., Settle, G. et al. (1991). Smell and taste disorders. A study of 750 patients from the University of Pennsylvania Smell and taste center. *Arch Otolaryngol Head Neck Surg*, Vol. 117:519-528.

Fokkens, WJ., Lund, VJ., Mullol, J et al. (2007). Position paper on Rhinosinusitis and Nasal Polyps 2007. *Rhinology* Suppl. Vol. 20:1-136.

Fairley, JW., Yardley, MPJ. & Durham, LH. (1993). Reliability and validity of a nasal symptom questionnaire for use as an outcome measure in clinical research and audit of functional endoscopic sinus surgery. *Clin Otolaryngol*, Vol. 18:436-437.

Giger, R., Dulguerov, P., Quinodoz, D. et al. (2004). Chronic panrhinosinusitis without nasal polyps: long-term outcome after functional endoscopic sinus surgery. *Otolaryngol Head Neck Surg*, Vol. 131:534-541.

Gill, TM. & Feinstein, AR. (1994). Acritical appraisal of the quality of life of quality-of-life measurements. *J Am Med Assoc*, Vol. 272:619-626.

Gliklich, RE. & Metson, R. (1995). The health impact of chronic sinusitis in patients seeking otolaryngologic care. *Otolaryngol Head Neck Surg*, Vol. 113:104-109.

Gliklich, RE. & Metson, R. (1995). Effect of sinus surgery on quality of life. *Otolaryngol Head Neck Surg*, Vol. 117:12-17.

Grammer, K., Fink, B. & Neave, N. (2005). Human pheromones and sexual attraction. *Eur J Obstet Gynecol Reprod Med*, Vol. 118:135-142.

Hai, PV., Lidstone, C. & Wallwork, B. (2010). The effect of endoscopic sinus surgery on bacterial biofilms in chronic rhinosinusitis. *Otolaryngol Head Neck Surg*, Vol. 142:27-32.

Havlicek, J., Murray, AK., Saxton, TK. et al. (2010). Current issues in the study of androstenes in human chemosignaling. *Vitam Horn*, Vol. 83:47-81.

Holbrook, E., Brown, C., Lyden, E. et al. (2005). Lack of significant correlation between rhinosinusitis symptoms and specific region of sinus CT scans. *Am J Rhinol*, Vol. 19:382-387.

Hopkins, C., Browne, JP., Slack, R. et al. (2006). The national comparative audit of surgery for nasal polyposis and chronic rhinosinusitis. Clin *Otolaryngol Allied Sci*, Vol. 31:390-399.

Hopkins, C., Browne, JP., Slack, R et al. (2007). The Lund-Mackay staging system for chronic rhinosinusitis: How is it used and what does it predict? *Otolaryngol Head Neck Surg*, Vol 137:555-561.

Hopkins, C., Gillett, S., Slack, R., Lund, VJ. &, Browne, JP. (2009). Psychometric validity of 22-item sinonasal outcome test. *Clin Otolaryngol*,Vol. 34:447-454.

Juniper, EF., Guyatt, GH., Willan, A. et al. (1994). Determining a minimal important change in disease-specific Quality of Life Questionnaire. *J Clin Epidemiol*, Vol. 47:81-87.

Ling, FT. & Kountakis, SE. (2007). Important clinical symptoms in patients undergoing functional endoscopic sinus surgery for chronic rhinosinusitis. *Laryngoscope*, Vol. 117:1090-1093.

Litvack, JR., Grieast, S., James, KE. et al. (2007). Endoscopic and Qualityy-of Life Outcomes After Revision Endoscopic Surgery. *Laryngoscope*, Vol. 117:2233-2238.

Litvack., JR., Mace, JC. & Smith, TL. (2009). Olfactory function and disease severity. *Am J Rhinol Allergy*, Vol.23:139-144.

Lund, VJ. (2001). Health related quality of life in sinonasal disease. *Rhinology*, Vol 39:182-186.

Lund, VJ., Black, JH., Szabó, LZ. et al. (2004). Efficacy and tolerability of budesonide aqueous nasal spray ich chronic rhinosinusitis patients. *Rhinology*, Vol. 42:57-62.

Kennedy DW. (1992). prognostic factores, outcomes, and staging in etmoid sinus surgery. *Laryngoscope*, Suppl 57:1-18.

Kirmaz, C., Aydemir, O., Bayrak, P. et al. (2005). Sexual dysfunction in patients with allergic rhinoconjuctivitis. *Ann Allergy Asthma Immunol*, Vol. 95:525-529.

Kountakis, SE, Arrango, P., Bradley Dewayne, et al. (2004). Molecular and cellular staging for the severity of chronic rhinosinusitis. *Laryngoscope*, Vol. 114:1895-1905.

Mace, JC., Michael, YL, Carlson, NC., et al. (2008). Effect of depression on quality of life improvement after endoscopic sinus surgery. *Laryngoscope*, Vol. 118:528-53

Mace, JC., Michael, YL, Carlson, NC., et al. (2010). Correlation between endoscopy score and quality of life changes after sinus surgery. *Arch Otolaryngol Head Neck*, Vol. 136:340-346.

Metson, R. & Gliklich, RE. (1998). Clinical outcome of endoscopic surgery for frontal sinusitis. *Arch Otolaryngol Head Neck Surg*, Vol. 124:1090-1096.

Miwa, T., Furukawa, M., Tsukatani, T et. al. (2001). Impact of olfactory impairment on quality of life and disability. *Arch Otolaryngol Head Neck Surg*, Vol. 127:497-503.

Morley, AD. & Sharp, HR. (2006). A review of sinonasal outcome scoring system- which is best? *Clinical Otolaryngology*, Vol. 31:103-109.

Naxakis, S., Athanasapoulos, I. & Vlastos I. (2009). Evaluation of nasal mucociliary clearance after medical or surgical treatment of chronic rhinosinusitis. *Eur Arch Otorhinolaryngol*. Vol. 266:1423-1426.

Piccirillo, JF., Merrit, MG. & Richards, ML. (2002). Psychometric and clinimetric validity of the 20-item Sino-Nasal Outcome Test (SNOT-20). *Otolaryngol Head Neck Surg*,Vol. 126:41-47.

Proimos, E., Papadakis, CE., Chimona D. et al. (2010). The effect of functional endoscopic sinus surgery on patients with asthma and CRS with nasal polyps. *Rhinology*, Vol. 48:331-338.

Ragab, SM., Lund, VJ., Scadding, G. et al. (2010). Impact of chronic rhinosinusitis therapy on quality of life; A prospective randomized controlled trial. *Rhinology*, Vol. 48:305-311.

Robinson, K., Gatehouse, S.& Browning, GG. (1996). Measuring patient benefit from otorhinolaryngological surgery and therapy. *Ann Otol Rhinol Laryngol*, Vol. 105:415-422.

Rudmik, L. & Smith, TL. (2011). Quality of life in patients with chronic rhinosinusitis. *Curr Allergy Asthma Rep*, Vol. 11:247-252.

Salhab, M, Matai, V, & Salam, MA. (2004). The impact of functional endoscopic sinus surgery on health status. *Rhinology*, Vol. 42:98-102.

Scadding, GK. & Williams, A. (2008) The burden of allergic rhinitis as reported by UK patients compared with their doctors. *Rhinology*, Vol. 46:99-105.

Schalek, P, Otruba, L. & Hahn, A. (2010). Quality of life in patients with chronic rhinosinusitis: A validation of the Czech version of SNOT-22 questionnaire. *Eur Arch Otorhinolaryngol*. Vol. 267:473-475.

Serrano, E., Neukirch, E., Pribil, C. et al. (2005). Nasal polyposis in France: impact on sleep and quality of life. *J Laryngol Otol*, Vol. 119:543-549.

Smith, TL., Batra, PS., Seiden, AM. et al. (2005). Evidence supporting endoscopic sinus surgery in the management of adult chronic rhinosinusitis: a systematic review. *Am J Rhinol*. Vol. 19:537-543.

Smith, TL., Litvack, JR, Hwang, PH. et al. (2010). Determinants of outcomes of sinus surgery: A Multi-Institutional prospective cohort study. *Otolaryngol Head Neck Surg*, Vol. 142:55-63.

Sobol, SE., Wright, ED. & Frenkiel, S. (1998). One-year outcome analysis of functional endoscopic sinus surgery for chronic sinusitis. *J Otolaryngol*, Vol. 27:252-257.

Soler, ZM., Mace, J. & Smith, TL. (2008). Symptom-based presentation of chronic rhinosinusitis and symptom specific outcomes after endoscopic sinus surgery. *Am J Rhinol*, Vol. 22:297-301.

Soler, ZM., Sauer, DA., Mace, J., et al. (2009). Relationship between clinical measures and histopathologic findings in chronic rhinosinusitis. *Otolaryngol Head Neck Surg*, Vol. 141:454-461.

Soler, ZM. & Smith, TL. (2010). Quality of life outcomes after functional endoscopic sinus surgery. *Otolaryngol Clin N Am*, Vol. 43:605-612.

Soler, ZM, Sauer, D., Mace, J. et al. (2010). Impact of mucosal eosinophilia and nasal polyposis on quality of life outcommes after sinus surgery. *Otolaryngol Head Neck Surg*, Vol. 142:64-71.

Suratt, PM, Turner, BL. & Wilhoit, SC. (1986). Effect of intranasal obstruction on breathing during the sleep. *Chest*, Vol. 90:324-329.

Temmel, AFP., Quint., C., Schickinger-Fischer, B. et al. (2002). Characteristics of olfactory disorders in relation to major causes of olfactory loss. *Arch Otolaryngol Head Neck Surg*, Vol. 128:635-641.

van Oene, CM., van Reij, EJF., Sprangers, MAG., Fokkens, WJ. (2007). Quality- assessment of disease-specific quality of life questionnaires for rhinitis and rhinosinusitis: a systematic review. *Allergy*, Vol.62:1359-1370.

Wabnitz, D., Nair, S. & Wormald, PJ. (2005). Correlation between preoperative symptom scores, quality of life questionnaires and staging with CT in patients chronic rhinosinusitis. *Am J Rhinol*, Vol. 19:91-96.

Ware, JE. & Sherbourne, CD. (1992). The MOS 36-Item Short Form Health Survey. I. Conceptual framework and item selection. *Med care*, Vol. 30, 473-483.

Wasan, A., Fernandez, E., Janison, RN. et al. (2007). Association of anxiety and depression with reported disease severity in patients undergoing evaluation for chronic rhinosinusitis. *Ann Otol Rhinol Laryngol*, Vol. 116:491-497.

Wilson, IB. & Clearly PD. (1995). Clinical variables with health-related quality of life. JAMA, Vol. 273:59-65.

Wright, ED. & Agrawal, S. (2007). Impact of perioperative systemic steroids on surgical outcomes in patients with chronic rhinosinusitis with polyposis: evaluation with a novel perioperative sinus endoscopy (POSE) scoring system. *Laryngoscope*, Suppl. 115:1-28.

Wyrwick, KW, Tierney, WM, Babu, AN. et al. (2005) A comparison of clinically important differences in health-related quality of life fore patients with chronic lung disease, asthma or heart disease. *Health Serv Res*, Vol. 40:577-592.

2

Microbiology Aspects of Rhinosinusitis

Agnieszka Magryś, Jolanta Paluch-Oleś and Maria Kozioł-Montewka
Department of Medical Microbiology, Medical University of Lublin, Poland

1. Introduction

Rhinosinusitis with its chronic benign course, failure in antibiotic treatment and acute exacerbations, usually require multiple courses of antibiotics or surgical procedures, or both. Nowadays, the pathogenic mechanisms of microbes in rhinosinusitis have gradually been revealed. Many current hypotheses focus on the formation of biofilms, bacterial superantigens, cytokine dysregulation, and abnormalities of cell-mediated immune responses (Kilty & Desrosiers, 2008; Zhang et al., 2005, Post et al., 2004).

"Rhinosinusitis" is a group of disorders characterized by inflammation of the mucosa of the nose and the paranasal sinuses. It is presently accepted that rhinosinusitis is initiated with an inflammatory insult (viral infection of upper respiratory tract, allergic rhinitis, etc.), followed by bacterial or fungal superinfection (Kennedy & Thaler, 1997; van Cauwenberge et al., 2006). Most upper respiratory tract infections are self-limited but progression to acute illness occurs and progression to chronic disease is common. Because specific treatment approaches are crucial for the different types of rhinosinusitis, this review focuses on microbiological aspects of rhinosinusitis.

2. Normal flora of upper respiratory tract

Most of the surfaces of the upper respiratory tract (including nasal and oral passages, nasopharynx, oropharynx, and trachea) are colonized by normal flora. The normal flora of human upper respiratory tract is harmless, and usually beneficial for the host. Two main functions are played by these bacteria, that are important in maintaining the healthy state of the host:

1. these organisms compete with pathogenic organisms for potential attachment sites,
2. they often produce substances (toxins or acids) which are bactericidal.

The nose is colonized predominantly by staphylococci, with *Staphylococcus aureus* and *Staphylococcus epidermidis* and diphtheroids as the leaders. The most important group of microorganisms native to oropharynx are also the alpha-hemolytic streptococci or viridans streptococci. This group includes *Streptococcus mitis, Streptococcus mutans, Streptococcus milleri,* and *Streptococcus salivarius*. It is believed that these bacteria act as antagonists against invasion by pathogenic streptococci.

But normal nasopharynx is not only the primary settlement of saprophytic bacteria. It is also the chief carrier of common respiratory pathogens, including *Streptococcus pneumoniae, Haemophilus influenzae* and *Moraxella catarrhalis* (Baron 1996).

3. Acute rhinosinusitis. Epidemiology and predisposing factors

3.1 Definition

Sinusitis is inflammation of the sinuses, which are air-filled cavities in the skull. This inflammation leads to blockade of the normal sinus drainage pathways (sinus ostia), which in turn leads to mucus retention, hypoxia, decreased mucociliary clearance, and predisposition to bacterial growth. Acute rhinosinusitis is an inflammatory condition involving the paranasal sinuses, as well as the lining of the paranasal passages, and it lasts up to 4 weeks, after which the symptoms resolve completely. Sinus infection is defined as the invasion and multiplication of microorganisms within a sinus. The etiology can be infectious (bacterial, viral, or fungal) or noninfectious (allergic) triggers (Fokkens et al., 2007; Thaler & Kennedy, 2008).

European Position Statement on Rhinosinusitis and Nasal Polyps defines acute rhinosinusitis as sudden onset of two or more symptoms, one of which should be either nasal blockade/obstruction/congestion or nasal discharge (anterior/posterior nasal dip) with facial pain/pressure or reduction or loss of smell (Fokkens et al., 2007).

3.2 Pathogenic factors of acute rhinosinusitis

Acute rhinosinusitis occurs when one of the mechanisms essential to sinus clearance breaks down. The ostiomeatal complex is particularly vulnerable to inflammatory changes, swelling and obstruction. Anatomic variations and other factors generally predispose patients to acute bacterial rhinosinusitis by causing inflammation in the ostiomeatal complex. Normal ciliary function, intact mucous membranes and normal mucous production are required for sinus clearance. Many factors can disturb these functional mechanisms predisposing to acute infection (Kennedy & Thaler, 1997; Anon, 2005; Fokkens et al., 2007).

The initial stages of rhinosinusitis comprise inflammatory swelling of the sinus epithelium and mucosa, secretion of proinflammatory factors, including cytokines, accumulation of inflammatory cells, such as eosinophils and lymphocytes, and obstruction of the sinus ostia (Hadley & Siegert, 2004).

Data shows that viral upper respiratory tract infections and pharyngeal colonization with group A streptococci predispose children to acute bacterial rhinosinusitis. The incidence of viral infections in acute rhinosinusitis is unknown, but it is estimated that 0.5-5% of viral infections lead to sinusitis (Brook et al., 2000; Fokkens et al., 2007).

Normal mucociliary flow is a key defense mechanism in the prevention of acute rhinosinusitis. Viral rhinosinusitis results in the loss of ciliated cells and mucociliary flow during the first week of infection. Consequently, the impaired mucociliary function during viral rhinosinusitis increases the risk of bacterial superinfection, which, in turn, results in further disruption of mucociliary flow (Fokkens et al., 2007; Sande & Gwaltney 2004). Exposure to bacterial toxins can also reduce ciliary function. Approximately 10% of cases of acute rhinosinusitis result from direct inoculation of the sinus with a large amount of bacteria. Bacterial infection causes inflammation and swelling, which leads to increased mucus production, reduced air flow through the nasal cavity and mucus congestion in the sinuses, enhancing bacterial growth (Hadley & Siegret, 2004).

Allergy is another factor that predispose to rhinosinusitis. Allergy can contribute to rhinosinusitis through either nasal congestion and subsequent ostial obstruction or direct allergic effects on sinus-lining cells. Obstructed sinus ostia, as the results of mucosal swelling and edema, may be more prone to infection **(Fokkens et al., 2007; Thaler & Kennedy, 2008).**

The other factors that predispose to acute rhinosinusitis are nasal polyposis, deviation of the nasal septum and dental procedures. Air pollution, cigarette smoking and overuse of topical decongestants impair ciliary action and predispose to rhinosinusitis as well (Fokkens et al., 2007).

3.3 Microbiology of acute rhinosinusitis: Viral or bacterial?

The upper respiratory tract represents a frequent site of infection because it is regularly exposed to direct contact and transmission of environmental pollutants and common microbes during breathing.

The most common factor associated with rhinosinusitis is upper respiratory infection, which is complicated by bacterial infection. Upper respiratory infections are mainly caused by viruses, leading to symptoms of common cold and inflammation of the paranasal sinuses. Viral rhinosinusitis has seasonal patterns of occurrence based on the virus involved. Rhinovirus is the most common cause of common cold and rhinosinusitis in all age groups, accounting for 30–70% of all respiratory illnesses. Other viruses causing upper respiratory infections are coronaviruses (7–18%), followed by influenza A and B, adenoviruses, parainfluenza viruses, respiratory syncytial viruses (RSV) and enteroviruses, all accounting for minor proportions of common cold cases (Thaler & Kennedy, 2008). Viral upper respiratory tract infection stimulates increases in inflammation and in the local immune response of the nasopharynx and surrounding mucosa. Some viruses, such as influenza virus, produce significant mucosal damage. Others promote the local production of cytokines and other inflammatory mediators, leading to the signs and symptoms of the common cold (Aanan, 2005). Clinically, patients experience a self-limiting illness lasting 3-7 days.

Acute bacterial rhinosinusitis complicates approximately 0.5% of adult and 5% pediatric cases of viral infections. It is usually a secondary infection resulting from ostiomeatal complex obstruction, impaired (delayed or absent) mucociliary clearance and weakened mucociliary integrity caused by an acute viral upper respiratory tract infection (Sande & Gwaltney, 2004).

Acute bacterial rhinosinusitis is a clinical condition characterized by nasal congestion, purulent rhinorrhea, postnasal dip and facial pain and pressure alone or with associated referred pain of the ears or teeth. The syndromes last for 7-14 days but no more than 4 weeks (Fokkens et al., 2007).

Several factors may predispose an individual with viral rhinosinusitis to acquire a secondary bacterial infection, including viral virulence, nosopharyngeal colonization and host immunity. The role of bacteria in acute rhinosinusitis is well defined. *Streptococcus pneumoniae* (20%-45%) and non typable strains of *Haemophilus influenzae* (22%-35%), are the most common pathogenic organisms in acute bacterial rhinosinusitis in adults. *Streptococcus pneumoniae* (30%-45%), non typable *Haemophilus influenzae* (20%-28%) and *Morraxella catarrhalis* (20-28%) are reported as predominant in children with acute bacterial rhinosinusitis. Until now *Staphylococcus aureus* has often been considered as a contaminant, but a recent data suggests that *Staphylococcus aureus* is a true pathogen in about 10% of cases of acute bacterial rhinosinusitis in adults (Benninger & Manz 2010; Payne, 2007) (Table 1). This is not surprising, as all these pathogens can be the parts of normal flora in upper respiratory tract.

The growing resistance to antimicrobial agents of all respiratory tract bacterial pathogens has made the management of bacterial rhinosinusitis more difficult.

Streptococcus pneumoniae are gram-positive, catalase-negative, facultatively anaerobic cocci that account for up to 45% of acute bacterial rhinosinusitis cases in adults and children. The rise of antimicrobial resistance in *Streptococcus pneumoniae* is a major concern. The most alarming situation is the occurrence of strains with decreased susceptibility to penicillin, that was the drug of choice in pneumococcal infections for many years. Penicillin resistance means the resistance or decreased susceptibility to other β-lactams. This is applied mostly for cephalosporins. Moreover, strains resistant to penicillin are also multi-drug resistant (resistance to macrolids, tetracycline, co-trimoxazole). However, they are still susceptible to increased doses of amoxicillin (Mazur, 2010; Aanan 2005).

Haemophilus influenzae is the second commonest agent of bacterial acute rhinosinusitis responsible for about 25% of rhinosinusitis cases in children. Studies have reported the presence of this bacterium in up to a third of adult rhinosinusitis patients as well. Beta-lactamase production is the mechanism of antimicrobial resistance for this organism. Of isolates from the paranasal sinus, 32.7% were found to be β-lactamase–positive. Other reports suggest a rate of 44%.

Moraxella catarrhalis is mainly isolated from children. Over 75% of all children harbor this bacterium, which causes about 25% of rhinosinusitis cases. The strains of *Moraxella catarrhalis* commonly (more than 90% strains) produce β-lactamases all over the world (Mazur, 2010; Aanan, 2005).

The widespread antibiotic resistance among pathogens that are agents of rhinosinusitis allows for the persistence of infection and the development of chronic rhinosinusitis (CRS) (Thaler & Kennedy, 2008).

Nowadays it is noted that the vaccination of children with heptavalent conjugate pneumococcal vaccine results in significant shift in causative pathogens of acute bacterial rhinosinusitis. While the proportion of *Streptococcus pneumoniae* declined by 11%, the proportion of *Haemophilus influenzae* increased by 6%. A small increase in the isolation of other pathogens (*Moraxella catarrhalis, Staphylococcus auresus* and *Streptococcus pyogenes*) was also noted (Brook et al., 2006). Widespread use of conjugate pneumococcal vaccine has led to decreasing incidence of pneumococcal acute bacterial rhinosinusitis, which may have implications for treatment recommendations for these infections (Benninger, 2008). This pathogen shift may also have an important effect on the severity of acute bacterial rhinosinusitis. It is documented, that patients with acute bactericidal rhinosinusitis infected with *Streptococus pneumoniae* have more significant symptoms and worse radiographic findings than those infected with *Haemophilus influenzae*. This fact could result in less severe symptoms and radiographic findings in patients with acute form of the disease (Benninger & Manz, 2010).

Pathogens	Percentages	
	Adults	Children
Viruses		
Rhinovirus	15%-40%	1%
Adenovirus	----	2%
Influenzae virus	5%	----
Parainfluenzae virus	3%	2%
Bacteria		
Streptococcus pneumoniae	20%-45%	30%-45%
*Haemophilus influenzae**	22%-35%	20%-28%
Moraxella catarrhalis	0%-8%	20%-28%
Staphylococcus aureus	0%-10%	0%-8%
Streptococcus pyogenes	0%-7%	3%-9%

* non typable strains

Table 1. The commonest pathogens in acute rhinosinusitis. Data are from (Thaler & Kennedy, 2008; Sande & Gwaltney, 2004).

3.4 Microbiology diagnostics of acute rhinosinusitis

Bacterial and viral rhinosinusitis are difficult to differentiate on clinical grounds. On the other hand, bacterial rhinosinusitis must be distinguished from viral infection and treated with antibiotics, because serious complications may be associated when bacterial superinfection develops. (Hytönen et al., 2000; Herrmann & Forsen 2004). The reference standard for the diagnosis of acute bacterial rhinosinusitis is sinus puncture with culture and recovery of bacteria in high density (≥ 10^4 colony forming units/mL) (Hart, 2007). Although sinus aspiration with the possible bacterial culture is the "gold standard" for the diagnosis of acute bacterial rhinosinusitis, it is not recommended in general practice. The reasons are that the procedure is invasive, time-consuming and potentially painful for the patient and can only be performed by a specialist as it requires a local anestethic. However, the results of sinus aspiration correlate with clinical and radiographic findings in patients with acute respiratory symptoms.

The most widely used diagnostic procedures for acute rhinosinusitis are signs and symptoms, supported by radiographic findings. Some experts believe that bacteriological cultures from the posterior parts of nasal cavity and nasopharyngeal aspirates best identify those patients with bacterial superinfection (Anan, 2005).

Because of the difficulty associated with distinguishing viral from bacterial rhinosinusitis, the diagnosis of acute bacterial rhinosinusitis is mostly reserved for patients who experience rhinosinusitis symptoms (eg, sinus pain, tooth pain, nasal congestion) for more than 7 days (Hart, 2007).

3.5 Current recommendations for diagnosing acute rhinosinusitis in children

Although sinus aspiration is the "gold standard" for the diagnosis of acute bacterial rhinosinusitis, it is not recommended method for routine diagnosis of bacterial sinus infections in children. According to recommendations of American Academy of Pediatrics the diagnosis of acute bacterial rhinusitis is based on clinical criteria in children who present with upper respiratory symptoms that are either persistent or severe (American Academy of Pediatrics, 2001).

Persistent symptoms are symptoms of upper respiratory tract infection that last longer than 10 days to 14 days, but less than 30 days. Such symptoms include nasal or postnasal discharge, daytime cough (which may be worse at night), or both.

Severe symptoms include a temperature of at least 39ºC and purulent nasal discharge present concurrently for at least 3 to 4 consecutive days in a child who seems ill. In this clinical presentation, the duration of symptoms is not important, and antimicrobial treatment is recommended to be started as soon as possible (American Academy of Pediatrics, 2001).

American Academy of Pediatrics has taken the position that, in children six years and younger who are at the peak age for developing acute bacterial sinusitis, a diagnosis can be made without performing imaging studies. However, controversy exists about the need for radiographs to confirm acute sinusitis in children older than six years with persistent symptoms and for children of any age with severe symptoms (American Academy of Pediatrics, 2001). The American College of Radiology recommends that the diagnosis be made on clinical criteria and that radiographs be used only in patients who do not recover or who worsen during the course of antimicrobial therapy (McAlister et al., 2000).

CT scans of the paranasal sinuses should be performed only when surgery is being considered. CT scans are indicated in children with complications of acute bacterial sinus infection or those with very persistent or recurrent infections that are not responsive to medical therapy (McAlister et al., 2000; American Academy of Pediatrics, 2001).

4. Chronic rhinosinusitis

4.1 Definition

Chronic rhinosinusitis can be defined as a group of disorders characterized by inflammation of the mucosal lining of the nasal cavity and para-nasal sinuses lasting for at least 12 weeks. Symptoms are much more subtle then with acute rhinosinusitis. In order to diagnose chronic rhinosinusitis, patients are required to have 2 of the following symptoms for at least 12 consecutive weeks: (1) anterior and /or posterior mucopurulent drainage, (2) nasal obstruction and (3) hyposmia or anosmia but also objective evidence of sino-nasal inflammation on both endoscopy and radiological imaging with computerised tomography. Fever is not typically observed. According to the definitions of the European Position Paper on Rhinosinusitis and Nasal Polyps, chronic rhinosinusitis and nasal polyposis are considered as one disease entity, in which nasal polyposis forms a subgroup of chronic rhinosinusitis (Fokkens et al., 2007).

Chronic rhinosinusitis is mostly diagnosed in association with predisposing conditions such as asthma, allergy, dental disease, cystic fibrosis, polyposis and immunodeficiency syndrome (Thaler & Kennedy, 2008; Kennedy & Thaler, 1997).

It has been postulated that chronic rhinosinusitis evolves from acute rhinosinusitis, but this has never been definitively proven. Also, the role of bacterial infection in chronic rhinosinusitis is less clear than in acute rhinosinusitis (Thaler & Kennedy, 2008).

4.2 Pathogenic factors

Chronic rhinosinusitis is now considered a multi-factorial disease involving multiple host and environmental factors. This factors has been broadly categorized into extrinsic or non-host related factors and intrinstic or host related factors. Extrinsic factors that have been implicated as etiologies contributing to the development of CRS include viral, bacterial, and/or fungal colonization and their associated pathogenicity (biofilms, superantigens, osteitis and non-IgE mediated eosinophilic inflammation) as well as exposure to inhaled substances, such as cigarette smoke or allergens. Intrinsic factors found to be associated with chronic rhinosinusitis include anatomic/structural abnormalities, genetic abnormalities, such as cystic fibrosis or primary ciliary dyskinesia and disorders in innate and cell mediated immune system (van Cauwenberg & van Hoeche, 2006).

The presence of intracellular *Staphylococcus aureus* in epithelial cells of the nasal mucosa has been suggested to play a significant risk for recurrent episodes of rhinosinusitis due to persistent bacterial clonotypes, which appear refractory to antimicrobial and surgical therapy (Plouin-Gaudon et al., 2006).

4.3 Bacteria and chronic rhinosinusitis

The microbiology of chronic rhinosinusitis differs when comparing to acute rhinosinusitis. Study shows that in patients with chronic rhinosinusitis, pathogens such as *Staphylococcus aureus*, coagulase negative streptococci and anaerobic Gram-negative bacteria replace the pathogens commonly found in bacterial acute rhinosinusitis. The prevalence of anaerobic species can be explained by physiologic changes in the sinuses including reduced oxygen tension and pH, thereby creating a favorable environment for these organisms (van Cauwenberge et al., 2006; Thaler & Kennedy 2008).

4.3.1 Controversy regarding the role of bacteria in chronic rhinosinusitis

In contrast with the well-established roles of microbes in the etiology of acute sinusitis with *Streptococcus pneumoniae, Moraxella catarrhalis* and non typable *Haemophilus influenzae* strains as the most common pathogens involved, the exact roles of all of these microbes in the etiology of chronic sinusitis are uncertain. Until now, there have been many controversies concerning the microbial involvement in chronic sinusitis (Kilty & Desrosiers, 2008; Thaler & Kennedy, 2008).

It has been postulated that in many cases of chronic rhinosinusitis bacteria can be present only as non-pathogens. This conclusion arose from the observation, that the sinuses are not sterile as once taught. Also, the fact that poor correlation is observed between clinical findings, microbiology and antibiotic therapy confirmed the limited role of bacteria in chronic rhinosinustis (Post et al., 2004; van Cauwenberge et al., 2006).

Much of the disagreement may be explained by methodology used. Different studies used different sampling methods as well as different methods to detect bacteria and quantify bacterial load (culture vs. PCR). It is thought that these differences may not only affect the culture yield rate but also the type of organism isolated (Kilty & Desrosiers, 2008).

Nowadays, the role of bacteria in chronic rhinosinusitis have gradually been revealed. Several theories raised to explain the patophysiology of this chronic disease. It is currently thought that chronic rhinosinusitis is an immunological inflammatory disease caused simultaneously or singly by several factors, such as: immune conditions, intrinsic upper airway factors, *Staphylococcus aureus* superantigens, and persistent biofilm presence and/or osteitis of the sinus wall (Bezerra et al., 2009). In this paper, the role of bacterial superantigens and biofilm will be overviewed.

4.3.2 Bacterial superantigens

The superantigen hypothesis of chronic rhinosinusitis suggests that bacterial toxins within the nose stimulate massive oligoclonal expansion of T-cell populations with subsequent eosinophil recruitment and tissue inflammation (Seiberling, Grammer, et al., 2005).

In the pathogenesis of chronic rhinosinusitis with nasal polyposis, this theory have been supported by several studies. Superantigens are microbial derived toxins capable of triggering massive T cell proliferation and activation. They have the ability to activate up to 30% of the T-cell population in contrast to the conventional antigen response, which activates only 0.01% of all T cells. In the acute setting superantigens may lead to the sudden and massive release of Th1 and Th2 cytokines which accounts for their acute toxicity (Llewelyn et al., 2002; Seiberling, Conley et al., 2005).

Evidence accumulates that *Staphylococcus aureus* colonizes a high percentage of patients with chronic rhinosinusitis with nasal polyposis. *Staphylococcus aureus* can secrete at least 19 different exotoxins capable of functioning as superantigens, triggering massive T-cell activation, and induces an overproduction of immunoglobulin E, as well as a severe possibly steroid-insensitive eosinophilic inflammation.(Zhang et al., 2005).

Understanding how superantigens overstimulate the immune system is crucial to set up rational therapeutics for chronic rhinosinusitis. Patients with eosinophilic chronic rhinosinusitis remain the most refractory to medical and surgical intervention (Seiberling, Conley et al., 2005).

4.3.3 Bacterial biofilm

One possible mechanism for the chronic nature of rhinosinusitis is the involvement of bacterial biofilms. Recent publications estimate that at least 65% of all chronic bacterial infections involve biofilms (Kilty & Desrosiers, 2008; Post et al., 2004).

Biofilms are three-dimensional bacterial aggregates embedded together in the slimelike matrix composed of polysaccharides, nucleic acids and proteins (extracellular polymeric substances). Bacteria in biofilm are under different transcriptional regulation and are thus phenotypically different than free living bacteria. The vast majority of bacteria, regardless of species, exist within a biofilm, including those that are important in rhinosinusitis, such as *Haemophilus influenzae, Streptococcus pneumoniae* and *Staphylococcus aureus* (Kilty & Desrosiers, 2008).

The formation of a bacterial biofilm occurs in several concurrent steps. The initiating event is the attachment of individual bacterial cells to a surface by weak reversible physical forces. Differentiation of the biofilm after attachment depends on cell-to-cell signaling, which facilitate the binding of other bacteria to the infected surface. This process initiates phenotypic changes within the bacteria to irreversibly secure the initial attachment.

The second stage involves irreversible attachment between specific microbial adhesins and the surface. One important element of this process is polysaccharide intracellular adhesion (PIA), that mediates the cell-cell interactions in some staphylococcal biofilms.

Cell aggregation into microcolonies and their division ensure the continued growth of the biofilm into complex structure. When biofilms reach their critical mass, single bacterium or aggregates of bacteria can disperse into the surrounding environment. After detachment bacteria can be redistributed to other areas of the host surface, where further biofilm growth can be initiated (Post et al., 2004).

Owing to its multicellular nature, biofilms provide bacteria with distinct advantages. An adventage that is extremely important clinically is that bacteria in biofilms are very resistant to antibiotics, capable of surviving antibiotic concentrations thousands of time greater than free living bacteria (Post et al., 2004). Also, biofilm formation makes the bacteria resistant to host defense mechanisms, because the aggregation of bacteria into biofilm cannot be phagocytized, humoral immune system is not effective against aggregated bacteria as well.

The same properties that make bacteria within biofilm resistant to antibiotics and to the attack of immune system also make it difficult to identify them in laboratory by routine methods. Bacterial biofilms have been found in patients with chronic rhinosinusitis by scanning electron microscopy (SEM), transmission electron microscopy (TEM), confocal scanning laser microscopy, or fluorescent in situ hybridization (FISH) successfully. The use of PCR-based techniques demonstrates a high detection rate of bacterial pathogens in chronic diseases when comparing with conventional culture technique (Kilty & Destrosiers, 2008).

The fact that bacterial existence in the form of biofilm in probably preferred in chronic infections, there is growing evidence for the presence of bacterial biofilms in chronic rhinosinusitis (Kilty & Desrosiers, 2008).

If bacterial biofilms are the cause of certain cases of chronic rhinosinusitis, then the treatment paradigms will have to be changed. Novel nonantimicrobial therapies may have clinical applications to prevent and destabilize biofilms.

5. References

Aanan, J.B. (2005). *Current management of acute bacterial rhinosinusitis and the role of moxifloxacin.* Clin. Infect. Dis. Vol. 41, pp. (S167-S176)

American Academy of Pediatrics: *Clinical Practice Guideline: Management of Sinusitis* (2001). Pediatrics, Vol. 108, pp. (798-808).

Baron, S. (1996). *Medical microbiology, 4th edition.* University of Texas Medical Branch at Galveston, ISBN – 10: 0-9631172-1-1, USA

Benninger, M.S. (2008). *Acute bacterial rhinosinusitis and otitis media: changes in pathogenicity following widespread use of pneumococcal conjugate vaccine.* Otolaryngol. Head Neck Surg. Vol. 138, No. 3, pp. 274-278

Benninger, M.S. & Manz R. (2010). The impact of vaccination on rhinosinusitis and otitis media. *Curr. Allergy Asthma* Rep. Vol. 10, pp. (411-418)

Bezerra, T.F.P., Padna, F.G., Gebrim, E.M.M.S., Saldiva, P.H.N. & Voegels, R.L. (2009). *Biofilms in chronic rhinosinusitis with nasal polyps.* Braz. J. Otolaryngol. Vol. 75, No. 6, pp. (788-793)

Brook, I., Foote P.A. & Hausfeld J.N. (2006). *Frequency of recovery of pathogens causing acute maxillary sinusitis in adults before and after introduction of vaccination of children with the 7-valent pneumococcal vaccine. J.* Med. Microbiol. Vol. 55, No. 7, pp. (943-946)

Brook, I., Gooch, W.M., Jenkins, S.G., Pichichero, m.E., Reiner, S.A. & Yamauchi T. (2000). *Medical management of acute bacterial sinusitis recommendations of a clinical advisory committee on pediatric and adult sinusitis.* Ann Otol Rhinol Laryngol Vol.109, pp. (1-20)

Fokkens, W.J., Lund, V.J., Mullol, J et al. (2007). *European Position Paper on Nasal Polyps.* Rhinology Vol. 45, Suppl. 20, pp. (1-139)

Hadley, J.A. & Siegret R. (2004). *Clinician's manual on rhinosinusitis.* Science Press Ltd, ISBN 1-85873-994-2, Italy

Hart, A.M. (2007). *Diagnosis and management of acute respiratory infections: acute rhinosinusitis.* J. Nurs. Pract. Vol.3, No.9, pp. (607-611)

Herrmann, BW & Forsen, JW Jr (2004) *Simultaneous intracranial and orbital complications of acute rhinosinusitis in children.* Int J Pediatr Otorhinolaryngol Vol. 68, No. 5, pp. (619–625)

Hytönen, M., Atula, T. & Pitkäranta, A. (2000) *Complications of acute sinusitis in children.* Acta Otolaryngol Suppl 543, pp.(154–157)

Kennedy, D.W. & Thaler E.R. (1997). Acute vs. chronic sinusitis: etiology, management, and outcomes. Infect. *Dis. Clin. Pract* Vol. 2 Suppl 2, pp. (S 49-S 58)

Kilty, S.J., & Desrosiers, M.Y. (2008). The role of bacterial biofilms and the pathophysiology of chronic rhinosinusitis. Curr. Allergy Asthma Rep. Vol. 8, pp.(227-233)

Llewelyn, M. & Cohen, J. (2002). Superantigens: microbial agents that corrupt immunity. Lancet Infect Dis. Vol. 2, No. 3, pp. (156-162)

Mazur, E. (2010). Rational antibiotic therapy of acute upper respiratory tract infections. *Pol. Merk. Lek.* XXIX, Vol. 173, pp. (304-308)

McAlister, W.H., Parker, B.R., Kushner, D.C. (2000). *Sinusitis in the pediatric population.* In: ACR Appropriateness Criteria. Reston, VA: American College of Radiology.

Payne, S.C, & Benninger, M.S. (2007). *Staphylococcus aureus is a major pathogen in acute bacterial rhinosinusitis: a meta-analysis.* Clin. Infect. Dis. Vol.45, pp. (121–127)

Plouin-Gaudon, I., Clement, S., Huggler, E , Chaponnier, C, Francosis, P., Lew, D., Schrenzel, J, Vaudaux, P. & Lacroix, J.S. (2006). *Intracellular residency is frequently associated with recurrent Staphylococcus aureus rhinosinusitis.* Rhinology. Vol. 44, No. 4, pp. (249-254)

Post, J.Ch., Stoodley, P., Hall-Stoodley, L. & Ehrlich, G.D. (2004). The role of biofilms in otolaryngologic infections. *Curr. Opin. in Otolaryngol. Head Neck Surg.*, Vol. 12, pp.(185-190)

Ryan, D. (2008). *Management of acute rhinosinusitis in primary care: changing paradigms and the role of intranasal corticosteroids.* Prim. Care Resp. J. Vol. 17, No. 3, pp. (148-155)

Sande, M.A. & Gwaltney, J.M. (2004). *Acute community-acquired bacterial sinusitis: continuing challenges and current management.* Clin. Infect. Dis. Vol. 39 Suppl 3, pp. (S151-S158)

Seiberling, K.A, Conley, D.B., Tripathi, A., Grammer, L.C., Shuh L, Haines, G.K., Schleimer, R.& Kern, R.C. (2005). *Superantigens and chronic rhinosinusitis: detection of staphylococcal exotoxins in nasal polyps.* The Laryngoscope, Vol. 115, pp. (1580-1585)

Seiberling, K.A., Grammer, L. & Kern, R.C. (2005). *Chronic rhinosinusitis and superantigens.* Otolaryngol. Clin. North Am. Vol. 38, No. 6, pp. (1215-1236)

Thaler, E.R. & Kennedy D.W. (2008). *Rhinosinusitis: a guide for diagnosis and management.* Springer. ISBN: 978-0-387-73061-5, USA.

van Cauwenberge, P, van Hoecke, H. & Bachert C. (2006) Pathogenesis of chronic rhinosinusitis. Curr. *Allergy Asthma Rep.* Vol. 6, pp. (487-494)

Zhang, N., Gevaert, P., van Zele, T. Perez-Novo, C., Patou, J., Holtapplers, G., van Cauvenberge, P. & Bachert C. (2005) An update on the impact of Staphylococcus aureus enterotoxins in chronic sinusitis with nasal polyposis. Rhinology. Vol. 43, No.3, pp. (162-168).

3

Chronic Rhinosinusitis and Olfactory Dysfunction

Huart Caroline[1,2], Franceschi Daniel[3] and Rombaux Philippe[1,2]
[1]*Department of Otorhinolaryngology, Cliniques Universitaires Saint-Luc, Brussels,*
[2]*Institute of Neuroscience, Université Catholique de Louvain, Brussels,*
[3]*Department of Otorhinolaryngology, Clinique Sainte-Elisabeth, Brussels,*
Belgium

1. Introduction

Chronic rhinosinusitis (CRS) is defined, according to the European Position Paper on Rhinosinusitis and Nasal Polyps (Fokkens et al., 2007), as "presence of two or more symptoms one of which should be either nasal blockage/obstruction/congestion or nasal discharge (anterior/posterior nasal drip) +/- facial pain/pressure +/- reduction or loss of smell for >12 weeks". Olfactory disorder thus appears to be one of the diagnosis criteria for CRS with or without nasal polyposis, underlining the importance of this specific symptom among patients with CRS. Inversely, CRS appears to be the most common cause of olfactory dysfunction in patients presenting to smell evaluating centers and account for 14-30% of the cases (Holbrook and Leopold, 2006; Landis et al., 2004; Mott and Leopold, 1991; Raviv and Kern 2004; Seiden and Duncan, 2001). What underlines the intimate connection between CRS and olfactory dysfunction.

Several studies have shown that the quality of life is severely impaired in patients suffering from olfactory disorders (Frasnelli and Hummel, 2005; Neuland et al., 2011). It is thus important to detect this symptom and to provide an optimal treatment to patients. Nowadays, we have medical and surgical treatments that may relieve patients but these results are still hazardous.

Good management and good support to patients highly depend on a good knowledge of this entity. We will thus review important issues about CRS and olfactory dysfunction, beginning with generalities about olfactory dysfunction, to continue with pathophysiology of this entity, assessment of olfactory function in patients, the contribution of imaging and finally effects of current treatments on olfactory function.

2. Olfactory dysfunction

The incidence of olfactory dysfunction among the population is still a matter of debate. Authors report an incidence of 1-3% of dysfunction among population (Hoffman et al., 1998; Murphy et al., 2002). Nevertheless a recent study by Landis et al. (2004) reported higher values of olfactory dysfunction among population without sinonasal complaints, with a rate of 4.7% of anosmia and 16% of hyposmia. The most common causes of olfactory disorder are CRS, upper respiratory tract infection and head trauma. It is also mandatory to note that in a significant number of cases the cause of olfactory dysfunction remains unknown, even after investigations. (Table 1)

1	Rhinosinusitis
2	Post upper respiratory tract infection
3	Idiopathic
4	Post traumatic
5	Iatrogen
6	Toxic
7	Congenital
8	Miscellaneous

Table 1. Etiologies of olfactory dysfunction listed in descending order. Rhinosinusitis appears to be the most important cause of olfactory dysfunction in the general population.

In the literature, CRS is described as the most common cause of olfactory dysfunction, accounting for 14-30% of cases (Holbrook and Leopold 2006; Mott and Leopold, 1991; Raviv and Kern 2004; Seiden and Duncan, 2001). Inversely, olfactory impairment is a common symptom affecting 61-83% of patients with CRS (Bhattacharyya, 2003; Litvak et al., 2008; Orlandi and Terrell, 2002; Soler et al., 2008). Nevertheless up to one quarter of patients with CRS are unaware of their decreased olfactory abilities, probably because the olfactory dysfunction in CRS develops slowly and in consequence only a few patients note this disorder (Nordin et al., 1995). Psychophysical tests results show that patients with CRS have quantitative disorders, between hyposmia and anosmia (Holbrook and Leopold 2006; Mott and Leopold, 1991; Raviv and Kern 2004; Seiden and Duncan, 2001; Welge-Luessen, 2009) and may report fluctuating symptoms (Apter et al., 1999). Also it is widely known that patients with CRS with polyps have a higher incidence of smell symptoms and anosmia than patients with CRS without polyps (Hellings and Rombaux, 2009).

Some studies have described that the severity of quantitative disorders is related to the importance of the sinonasal disease (Litvack et al., 2008, 2009a). Indeed, the mean endoscopy score and the mean CT score are significantly higher (more abnormal) in patients with hyposmia and anosmia than in patients with normosmia (Litvack et al., 2009a). Also, the opacification of the olfactory cleft on the CT scan seems to have a negative correlation with the olfactory function (Chang et al., 2009).

Patients with CRS not only report quantitative olfactory dysfunction but also qualitative dysfunction such as parosmia and phantosmia. However, these symptoms seem less frequent when related to sinonasal disease than to other etiologies (i.e. post-infectious, post traumatic) and Reden et al. (2007) reported incidence of parosmia and phantosmia in patients with CRS of 28% and 7%, respectively.

It is also mandatory to note that the quality of life of patients suffering from olfactory disorders is severely impaired. Indeed it has been described that patients with olfactory disorders not only complain about daily life problems (cooking, detection of potentially dangerous odors) (Temmel et al., 2002) but also have a higher prevalence of mild to severe depression compared to the general population (Deems et al., 1991). Using questionnaire of olfactory disorder and psychometric tests some authors reported that patients suffering from quantitative olfactory impairment significantly more complaints that patients with normosmia and this was even more important if they had associated parosmia (Frasnelli and Hummel, 2005; Neuland et al., 2011). Finally, since patients reporting an improvement of their olfactory abilities have a better quality of life than patients reporting no improvement (Miwa et al., 2001); it is essential to investigate about the etiology of olfactory dysfunction in instance to provide an optimal treatment to the patients. Particularly in cases of chronic rhinosinusitis, different treatments are available and improve olfactory function. They will be discussed later.

3. Pathophysiology

Traditionally, olfactory dysfunction in CRS is explained by a conductive olfactory loss, caused by swollen or hypertrophic nasal mucosa or nasal polyps, inducing an impaired access of odorants to the olfactory cleft. But clinical studies have failed to prove this hypothesis, as there is only little correlation between nasal resistance and the degree of olfactory dysfunction (Doty and Frye, 1989; Cowart et al., 1992). In addition, results of surgical therapy, although improving the nasal patency, are sometimes uncertain when considering the olfactory dysfunction.

Some studies have shown that the olfactory disturbance might also be explained by inflammatory process in the olfactory cleft (Konstantinidis et al., 2007). Indeed, biopsies of the olfactory neuroepithelium in patients suffering from CRS revealed inflammatory changes in the nasal mucosa and apoptotic pathological changes, including the olfactory receptor neurons and olfactory supporting cells (Hellings and Rombaux, 2009; Naessen, 1971). Also, inflammatory cells release inflammatory mediators, which are known to trigger hypersecretion in respiratory and Bowman's glands (Hellings and Rombaux, 2009; Getchell and Mellert, 1991; Downey et al., 1996). Hypersecretion of Bowman's gland is thought to alter the ion concentrations of olfactory mucus, affecting the olfactory transduction process (Kern et al., 1997; Joshi et al., 1987). In addition, cytokines and mediators, particularly those released by eosinophils, may be toxic to olfactory receptor neurons (Apter et al., 1992; Nakashima et al, 1985), and the degree of inflammation changes in the neuropithelium is related to the severity of olfactory dysfunction (Kern, 2000)

Patients with nasal polyps show a higher incidence of olfactory disturbances and a higher incidence of anosmia than patients with CRS without polyps. This more severe symptomatology may be explained by the conductive olfactory loss induced by polyps but also by degenerative changes associated with recurrent infections, scaring, chronic nasal medication, exotoxins and enhanced secretion of cytokines from Staphylococcus Aureus infection and neurotoxic cytokines released by a huge eosinophilic population (Bernstein et al., 2011; Holcomb et al., 1996; Joshi et al., 1987; Litvack et al., 2008; Vento et al., 2001; Wang et al., 2010).

4. Assessment of olfactory function

Assessment of olfactory function should be considered in the clinical evaluation of patients suffering from chronic rhinosinusitis and complaining of olfactory disorders. Not only this evaluation allows detecting and quantifying olfactory disorders but also it is useful to objectively and reproducibly assess the efficacy of a treatment on olfactory function.

Odorants can reach the olfactory cleft both orthonasally (from the nostrils to the olfactory cleft) and retronasally (from the oral cavity to the olfactory cleft).

The most widely used tests for the evaluation evaluation of the orthonasal function are the Sniffin' Sticks test (Hummel et al., 2007; Burghart Medical Technology, Wedel, Germany) and the UPSIT (University of Pennsylvania smell identification test) (Doty et al., 1984). These semi-objective tests have the advantage of being easy to implement and of having been validated in multicenter studies. The Sniffin' Sticks test consists in felt-tip pens that are presented in front of the nose of the patient. It encompasses three different approaches. First the odor threshold (T) assessment; second the odor discrimination (D) and third odor identification (I). To judge the olfactory function, these three results are added together to provide a total TDI score. The UPSIT test 40 items. It encompasses fours "scratch and sniff" booklets that can be self administrated or applied by a third party. Odorants are embedded in microcapsules positioned on brown strips at the bottom of the page of booklets. The stimuli are released by scratching the strip with a pencil and subjects have to choice one of the four proposed descriptors that best corresponds to odor (Doty et al., 1984; Tourbier and Doty, 2007). These two tests are forced choice, what mean that the subject must provide a response even if no odor is perceived.

Retronasal olfactory performances can also be evaluated following a standardized method using a row of 20 items. Powder substances are applied using squeezable plastic vials in the middle of the tongue inside the oral cavity. Each substance is identified by means of a forced-choice procedure between 4 items. (Heilmann et al., 2002)

Nevertheless these tests have the disadvantage to be semi-objective and might be biased by the patient's response.

The objective evaluation of the olfactory function relies on event-related potentials technique. This technique is based on the fact that brief olfactory stimulus elicit transient changes in the ongoing electrographic activity. To evaluate olfactory function a pure odorant substance (i.e. 2-phenylethanol) is delivered in the nose of the patients (Kobal and Hummel, 1988). Since the magnitude of the transient olfactory-induced EEG deflection is much smaller than the magnitude of the background EEG, the event is repeated several times and recorded responses are the added and averaged into a single waveform to increase the signal to noise ratio. The bulk of olfactory chemosensory event-related potentials consist of a negative component (N1) occurring between 320 and 450 ms after stimulus onset, followed by a positive (P2) component occurring between 530-800 ms (Hummel et al., 1992; Hummel et al., 2003; Hummel and Kobal, 1999, 2002; Rombaux et al., 2006).

In cases of chronic rhinosinusitis, both orthonasal and retronasal scores can be decreased, with scoring of both anosmia and hyposmia. Electrophysiological investigations show abnormal responses with in moderate cases decreased amplitude and an increased latency and in severe cases the absence of olfactory responses (Rombaux et al., 2009). It is interesting to note that while in chronic rhinosinusitis, there is no difference between orthonasal and retronasal score, patients with CRS with polyps have a better retronasal than orthonasal score (Landis et al., 2003). Moreover ortho- and retronasal scores do not have a correlation when patient demonstrate an olfactory dysfunction related to sinonasal disease score proving that ortho- and retronasal scores have a distinct evolution in such cases (Rombaux et al., 2008).

5. Imaging of the olfactory apparatus in CRS

The MRI is the imaging modality of choice for the evaluation of the olfactory apparatus since it allows examining the olfactory bulb, olfactory tract and central olfactory projection areas. The assessment of olfactory bulb volume is particularly useful in the evaluation of olfactory disorder associated with CRS. Rombaux et al. (2008) demonstrated that the olfactory bulb volume is correlated with the sinonasal disease score, and patients having a sinonasal disease score > or = 12 significantly have larger olfactory bulb volume than patients with higher score. Smaller olfactory bulb volume is thus associated with a higher degree of sinonasal pathology. On contrast the olfactory function of the patients assessed with psychophysical testing was only slightly decreased or was even normal, emphasizing the idea that the olfactory bulb volume changes are more sensitive to subtle changes in the olfactory system than results of psychophysical testing. (Figure1)

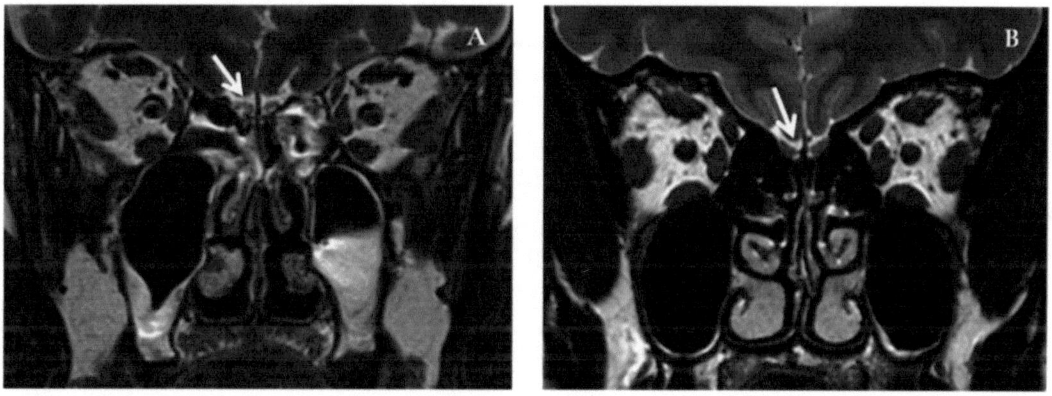

Fig. 1. T2-MRI on the coronal place of patient suffering from CRS (A) and control subject (B). Note that the olfactory bulb (white arrow) of the patient seems smaller than the OB of the control subject.

CT scan can also be useful in the assessment of patients with olfactory dysfunction associated with CRS. Litvack et al. (2009a) have shown that the severity of quantitative olfactory disorder is associated with the importance of the sinonasal disease and that mean CT score is significantly higher in patients with hyposmia and anosmia than in normosmic patient. It was also demonstrated that the opacification of the olfactory cleft has a negative correlation with the olfactory function in patients with CRS and that it is significantly correlated with the postoperative olfactory results; patients with mild opacification having better postoperative results than patients with moderate and severe anterior olfactory cleft result (Kim et al., 2011).

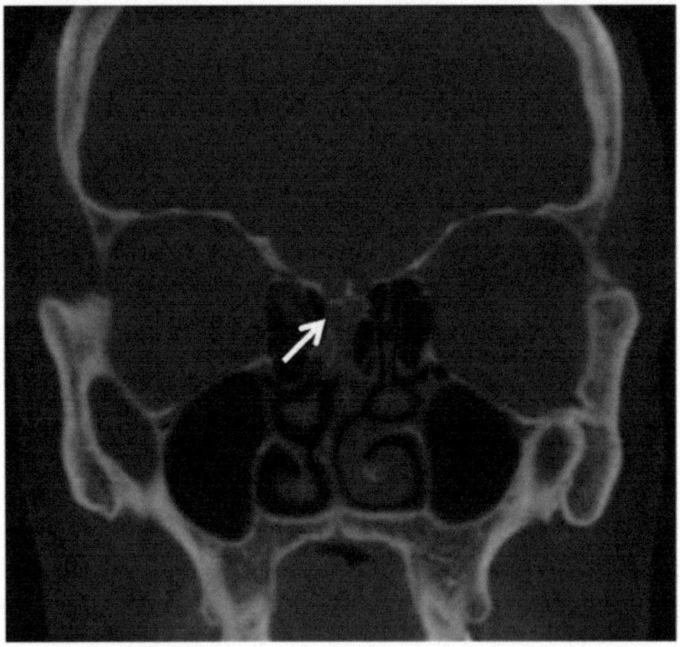

Fig. 2. CT-Scan in the coronal plane of a patient suffering from quantitative olfactory disorder. We can note on this picture an opacification of the olfactory cleft (white arrow) whereas there is no obvious rhinosinusitis. This image represents a so-called "olfactory cleft disease".

6. Predictors of olfactory dysfunction in patients with CRS

As we discuss previously, it is agreed that the severity of olfactory dysfunction is related to the importance of the sinonasal disease (Litvack et al., 2008, 2009a) and that the mean endoscopy and mean CT score are significantly higher in patients with hyposmia and anosmia than in normosmic patients (Litvack et al., 2009a).

But common comorbidities have also been incriminated as severity factors of olfactory loss related to the CRS. Some authors have incriminated age of patients, smoking status, nasal polyposis, asthma, allergic rhinitis, previous endoscopic sinus surgery, septal deviation and inferior turbinate hypertrophy to cause olfactory dysfunction but the results are conflicting (Apter et al., 1999; Damm et al., 2003; Doty and Mishra, 2001; Kimmelman, 1994; Litvack et al., 2008; Simola and Malmberg, 1998). Nevertheless, the majority of authors agree that the age of patients and the presence of nasal polyps are predictors of olfactory dysfunction in CRS (Apter et al., 1999; Doty and Mishra, 2001; Litvack et al., 2008; Simola and Malmberg, 1998). Nasal polyposis is a significant predictor of olfactory dysfunction and it has been showed that there is a negative correlation between the size of the nasal polyps and the olfactory performance. Also, in patients with nasal polyposis, the blood eosinophilia seems to be correlated with subjective smell reduction (Hox et al., 2010).

On contrast, studies agree that semi-objective olfactory testing are not correlated with disease-specific or general health-related quality of life instruments (Litvack et al., 2009a; Hox et al., 2010)

7. Effects of treatment on olfactory function

7.1 Medical therapy and smell dysfunction

Only a few clinical studies have been conducted dealing with the improvement of olfactory function as a primary outcome in sinonasal disease treatment. Clinical trials of medical treatment for smell disorders associated with CRS have evaluated the efficacy of nasal and oral corticosteroid treatment, but we found no studies about other treatments that are currently used in the treatment of CRS (antileukotrienes, antihistamines,…).

Corticosteroids with their potent anti-inflammatory effects are admitted to be the standard treatment for olfactory disorders induced by CRS. Their action mechanism on olfactory function might be explained by an inhibition of the release of proinflammatory mediators (i.e. cytokines, adhesion molecules, mast cells, basophiles, eosinophiles) and a reduction in mucosa swelling (Demoly, 2007; Mygind et al., 2001).

Following EPOS recommendations, nasal steroids are recommended as the first line treatment for CRS with or without nasal polyps (Fokkens et al., 2007). Studies have evaluated the efficacy of different topical corticosteroids such as Betamethasone, Flunisolide, Mometasone Furoate, Fluticasone Propionate, Budesonide, Beclomethasone. Studies show that these drugs appear to be highly effective for most of the symptoms associated with CRS, including smell disorder, with a rapid onset of action and a cumulative effect after several days of use. In addition, they have the advantage of being a local therapy with limited side effects. Nevertheless the improvement in olfaction is frequently transient and incomplete (Blomqvist et al., 2003; Golding-Wood et al., 1996; Hellings and Rombaux, 2009; Lildholdt et al., 1995; Mott et al., 1997; Stuck et al., 2003).

Oral steroids are recommended in the treatment of CRS with nasal polyps as a second line treatment (Fokkens et al, 2007). Several studies have investigated the efficacy of oral steroids in patients with CRS with or without polyps. They have shown that these potent anti-inflammatory drugs increase the olfactory function and they appear to be more effective than nasal steroids (Heilmann et al., 2004; Vaidyanathan et al., 2011). Moreover, an initial oral steroid therapy followed by topical steroid therapy seems to be more effective than topical steroid therapy alone (Vaidyanathan et al., 2011). Nevertheless oral steroids have important side effects if they are frequently administrated or if their administration is prolonged. Bonfils et al. (2006) evaluated the risk of oral steroid treatment in patients with CRS with nasal polyps and showed that almost 50% of patients who received more than three short courses of oral steroid treatment had an asymptomatic adrenal insufficiency. Oral corticosteroids should thus be prescribed only if necessary and should be avoided if possible.

7.2 Surgical therapy and smell dysfunction

Functional endoscopic sinus surgery (FESS) is widely accepted as a treatment for chronic rhinosinusitis with or without nasal polyps after failure of the medical therapy.

The only randomized study to attempt comparison between steroid therapy and polypectomy showed significant improvement of subjective and objective olfactory function in both groups, remaining for one year. However these results should be tempered by the fact that the smell evaluation methodology was not described (Lildholdt, 1989)

Several studies have investigated the effect of FESS on olfactory function (for a review see Bonfils et al., 2009). Nevertheless the literature shows that there are major variations in the selection of patients for the surgery and some studies have poor validity because of poorly defined patient groups, lack of clear inclusion or exclusion criteria, poor description of the surgical procedure and poor description of the olfactory evaluation tool.

In this literature, olfactory function was assessed either by subjective patient self-reported olfactory function or by semi-objective olfactory testing (i.e. UPSIT). Considering patients self reported olfactory function, authors agree that FESS lead to a significant improvement of olfactory dysfunction. Park et al. (1998) showed that olfactory disturbance was reported in 72% of patients with CRS with or without polyps or recurrent acute rhinosinusitis preoperatively compared with 38% following FESS. Lund and Mac Kay (1994) also reported that 79% of patients reported improved olfaction after FESS. Klossek et al. (1997) reported a series of patients with nasal polyposis. 100% of patients had anosmia pre-operatively while after surgery 78% of patients recovered the sense of smell. Levine et al. (1990) reported a series of 250 patients with CRS with or without nasal polyps and noted only 16% of patients complaining of smell disturbance before surgery and 3% patients reporting anosmia after a mean follow-up of one year after surgery. Jakobsen and Svendstrup (2000) reported a series of 237 patients with CRS with or without nasal polyps. Anosmia was present in 48% of the patients with nasal polyps before surgery against 21 % after surgery. Only few studies have investigated the effect of FESS on olfactory function by using semi-objective olfactory testing. They have also shown that FESS as a significant positive effect on olfactory function. For examples, Lund and Scading (1994) evaluated olfactory function of patients with CRS using UPSIT and showed significant UPSIT score improvement after surgery. Downey et al. (1996) also used UPSIT to assess the olfactory function of patients with CRS pre- and post-operatively and showed that after surgery, 52% of patients had higher UPSIT score. Min et al. (1995) tested olfactory thresholds to butanol in patients with CRS. Before surgery, 33 % of patients had anosmia and 45% of patients had hyposmia. After surgery these percentages were 16% and 46% respectively. Delank and Stoll (1998) noted a post operative improvement of olfactory function assessed by olfactory thresholds and discrimination in 70% of patients with CRS. Klimek et al. (1997) reported improved odor identification and discrimination score after FESS in patients with CRS with nasal polyps. Hence, FESS seems to significantly improve olfactory function in patients with CRS with or without polyps.

Gudziol et al. (2009) explored the influence of the treatment of CRS on the olfactory function. They measured olfactory bulb volume and olfactory function of patients suffering from CRS before treatment and 3 months after. They showed that the olfactory bulb volume significantly increases after treatment and that the increase of olfactory bulb volume correlated significantly with an increase in odor thresholds.

Some authors have also studied the correlation between the severity of CRS and surgical outcomes on olfaction. It was reported that the improvement after FESS is significantly better in patients with severe olfactory dysfunction whereas it is not in patients with mild olfactory dysfunction (Litvack et al., 2009b, Soler et al., 2010). The degree of nasal obstruction, the extent of the rhinosinusitis disease (evaluate by symptom score or CT scan), the coexistence of nasal polyps or allergic rhinitis do not predict the possibility of olfactory improvement after FESS (Bhattacharyya, 2006; Jiang et al., 2009; Wright and Agrawal, 2007). In addition, Jankowski et al. (Jankowski and Bodino, 2003) demonstrated that there was a correlation between the improvement of subjective olfactory function after oral corticosteroids given preoperatively and olfactory function 1 year after nazalisation.

Jankowski et al. (1997) compared the impact of different surgical approaches on olfactory function. Olfaction was evaluated by a 10-point visual analogue scale. They reported that improvement of olfaction was similar in both functional ethmoidectomy group and radical ethmoidectomy group six months after surgery. Nevertheless olfaction decreased in the functional ethmoidectomy group after six months while it was stable in the radical ethmoidectomy group.

8. Conclusion

CRS is the major cause of olfactory dysfunction among the population. The exact pathophysiology is this entity is still unclear. The olfactory dysfunction in these patients is reversible, as proved by the effect of treatments and MRI studies. Nevertheless, most studies show that the improvement of olfactory function is usually transient and incomplete. Different causes are hypothesized, but this is still a matter of debate. Future studies are necessary to better understand this entity.

9. References

Apter AJ, Gent JF & Frank ME (1999). Fluctuating olfactory sensitivity and distorted odor perception in allergic rhinitis. *Arch Otolaryngol Head Neck Surg,* 125 (9):1005-10

Apter AJ, Mott AE & Cain WS (1992). Olfactory loss and allergic rhinitis. *J Allergy Clin Immun,* 90:670-680

Bernsteins JM, Allen C, Rich G, Dryja D, Bina P, Reiser R, Ballow M & Wilding GE (2011). Further observations on the role of Staphylococcus Aureus exotoxins and IgE in the pathogenesis of nasal polyposis. *Laryngoscope,* 121(3):647-55

Bhattacharyya N (2003). The economic burden and symptom manifestations of chronic rhinosinusitis. *Am J Rhinol,* 17:27-32

Bhattacharyya N (2006). Radiographic stage fails to predict symptom outcomes after endoscopic sinus surgery for chronic rhinosinusitis. *Laryngoscope,* 116(1):18-22

Blomqvist EH, Lundblad L, Bergstedt H & Stjärne P (2003). Placebo-controlled randomized, double-blind study evaluating the efficacy of fluticasone propionate nasal spray for the treatment of patients with hyposmia/anosmia. *Acta Otolaryngol,* 123:862-868

Bonfils P, Halimi P & Malinvaud D (2006). Adrenal suppression and osteoporosis after treatment of nasal polyposis. *Acta Otolaryngol,* 126(11): 1195-1200

Bonfils P, Malinvaud Y, Soudry Y, Devars du Maine M & Laccourreye O (2009). Surgical therapy and olfactory function. *B-ENT,* 5 Suppl 13:77-87

Chang H, Lee HJ, Mo JH, Lee CH & Kim JW (2009). Clinical implication of the olfactory cleft in patients with chronic rhinosinusitis and olfactory loss. *Arch Otolaryngol Head Neck Surg,* 135(10):988-92

Cowart B, Flynn-Rodden K, McGeady S &Lowry LD (1992). Hyposmia in allergic rhinitis. *J Allergy Clin Immunol,* 9:747-751

Damm M, Eckel HE, Jungehulsing M &Hummel T (2003). Olfactory changes at threshold and suprathreshold levels following septoplasty with partial inferior turbinectomy. *Annals Otol Rhinol Laryngol,* 112:91-97

Deems DA, Doty RL, Settle RG, Moore-Gillon V, Shaman P, Mester AF, Kimmelman CP, Brightman VJ & Snow JB (1991). Smell and taste disorders: a study of 750 patients from the University of Pennsylvania Smell and Taste Center. *Arch Otolaryngol Head Neck Surg,* 117:519-528

Delank KW & Stoll W (1998). Olfactory function after functional endoscopic sinus surgery for chronic rhinoinusitis. *Rhinology,* 36:15-19

Demoly P (2008). Safety of intranasal corticosteroids in acute rhinosinusitis. *Am J Otolaryngol,* 29(6):403-13

Doty RL & Frye R (1989). Influence of nasal obstruction on smell function. *Otolaryngol Clin North Am,* 22:397-411

Doty RL & Mishra A (2001). Olfaction and its alteration by nasal obstruction, rhinitis and rhinosinusitis. *Laryngoscope,* 111:409-423

Doty RL, Shaman P & Dann M (1984). Development of the University of Pennsylvania Smell Identification Test: a standardized microencapsulated test of olfactory function. *Physiol Behav,* 32(3):489-502

Downey LL, Jacobs JB &Leibowitz RA (1996). Anosmia and chronic sinus disease. *Otolaryngol Head Neck Surg,* 115:24-28

Fokkens WJ, Lund VJ, Mullol J et al (2007). European Position Paper on Rhinosinusitis and Nasal Polyps 2007. *Rhinology Suppl,* 20:1-139

Frasnelli J & Hummel T (2005). Olfactory dysfunction and daily life. *Eur Arch Otorhinolaryngol,* 262(3):231-235

Getchell M & Mellert T (1991). Olfactory mucus secretion. In: *Smell and taste in health and disease.* Getchell TV, Bartoshuk LM, Doty RL, Snow J, eds, pp.83-95, Raven Press editor, ISBN-10:0881677981, New York

Golding-Wood DG, Holmstrom M, Darby Y, Scadding GK & Lund VJ (1996). The treatment of intranasal hyposmia with intranasal steroids. *J Laryngol Otol,* 110:132-135

Gudziol V, Buschhüter D, Abolmaali N, Gerber J, Rombaux P & Hummel T (2009). Increasing olfactory bulb volume due to treatment of chronic rhinosinusitis – a longitudinal study. *Brain,* 132 (Pt 11):3096-101

Heilmann S, Huettenbrink KB & Hummel T (2004). Local and systemic administration of corticosteroids in the treatment of olfactory loss. *Am J Rhinol,* 18:29-33

Heilmann S, Strehle G, Rosenheim K, Damm M & Hummel T (2002). Clinical assessment of retronasal olfactory function. *Acta Otolaryngol Head Neck Surg,* 128(4):414-8

Hellings PW & Rombaux P (2009). Medical therapy and smell dysfunction. *B-ENT,* 5 Suppl 13:71-5

Hoffman HJ, Ishii EK & MacTurk RH (1998). Age related changes in the prevalence of smell and taste problems among the United States adult population: results of the 1994 Disability Supplement to the National Health Interview Survey (NHIS). *Ann N Y Acad Sci,* 855:716-722

Holbrook EH & Leopold DA (2006). An updated review of clinical olfaction. *Curr Opin Otolaryngol Head Neck Surg,* 14:23-28

Holcomb JD, Graham S & Calof AL (1996). Neuronal homeostasis in mammalian olfactory epithelium: a review. *Am J Rhinol* 10(3):125-134

Hox V, Bobic S, Callebaux I, Jorissen M & Hellings PW (2010). Nasal obstruction and smell impairment in nasal polyp disease: correlation between objective and subjective parameters. *Rhinology,* 48(4):426-32

Hummel T & Kobal G (1999). Differences in human evokes potentials to trigeminal stimuli change in relation to the interval between repetitive stimulation of the nasal mucosa. *Eur Arch Otorhinolaryngol,* 256:16-21

Hummel T & Kobal G (2002). Olfactory event-related potentials. In: *Methods and New frontiers in Neurosciences,* Simon SA editor, pp. 123-148, CRC Press, Boca Raton

Hummel T, Futschik T, Frasnelli J & Hüttenbrink KB (2003). Effects of olfactory function, age, and gender on trigeminally mediated sensations: a study based on the lateralization of chemosensory stimuli. *Toxicol Lett,* 140-141:173-80

Hummel T, Kobal G, Gudziol H & Mackay-Sim A (2007). Normative data for the Sniffin Sticks including test of odor identification, odor discrimination and odor thresholds: an upgrade based on a group of more than 3000 subjects. *Eur Arch Otorhinol,* 264:237-243

Hummel T, Livermore A, Hummel C & Kobal G (1992). Chemosensory event-related potentials in man; relation to olfactory and painful sensations elicited by nicotine. *Electroencephalogr Clin Neurophysiol,* 84(2):192-5

Jakobsen J & Svendstrup F (2000). Functional endoscopic sinus surgery in chronic sinusitis - a series of 237 consecutively operated patients. *Acta Otolaryngol Suppl,* 543:158-161

Jankowski R & Bodino C (2003). Olfaction in patients with nasal polyposis: effects of systemic steroids and radical ethmoidectomy with middle turbinate resection (nazalisation). *Rhinology,* 41(4):220-30

Jankowski R, Pigret D & Decroocq F (1997). Comparison of functional results after ethmoidectomy and nazalisation for diffuse and severe nasal polyposis. *Acta Otolaryngol.* 117: 601-608

Jiang RS, Su MC, Liang KL, Shiao JY, Hsin CH, Lu FJ & Chen WK (2009). Preoperative prognostic factors for olfactory change after functional endoscopic sinus surgery. *Am J Rhinol Allergy,* 23(1):64-70

Joshi H, Getchell ML, Zielinski B & Getchell TV (1987). Spectrophotometric determination of cation concentrations in olfactory mucus. *Neurosci Lett,* 82 (3): 321-326

Kern RC, Foster JD& Pitovski DZ (1997). Glucocorticoid (type II) receptors in the olfactory mucosa of the guinea pig: RU 28362. *Chem sens,* 22:313-319

Kern RC. Chronic sinusitis and anosmia: pathologic changes in the olfactory mucosa. Laryngoscope 2000; 110(7):1071-7

Kim DW, Kim JY & Jeon SY (2011). The status of the olfactory cleft may predict postoperative olfactory function in chronic rhinosinusitis with nasal polyposis. *Am J Rhinol Allergy,* 25(2):90-4

Kimmelman CP (1994).The risk of olfaction from nasal surgery. *Laryngoscope,* 104:981-988

Klimek L, Moll B, Amedee RG & Mann WJ (1997). Olfactory function after microscopic endonasal surgery in patients with nasal polyps. *Am J Rhinol,* 11:251-255

Klossek JM, Peloquin L, Friedman WH, Ferrier JC & Fontanel JP (1997). Diffuse nasal polyposis: post-operative long-term results after endoscopic sinus surgery and frontal irrigation. *Otolaryngol Head Neck Surg.* 117:355-361

Kobal G & Hummel T (1988). Cerebral chemosensory evoked potentials elicited by chemical stimulation of the human olfactory and respiratory nasal mucosa. *Electroencephalogr Clin Neurophysiol,* 71:241-50

Konstantinidis I, Triaridis S, Printza A, Vital V, Ferekidis E & Constantinidis J (2007). Olfactory dysfunction in nasal polyposis: correlation with computed tomography findings. *ORL J Otorhinolaryngol Relat Spec,* 69(4):226-232

Landis BN, Giger R, Richchetti A, Leuchter I, Hugentobler M, Hummel T & Lacroix JS (2003). Retronasal olfactory function in nasal polyposis. *Laryngoscope,* 113(11):1993-7

Landis BN, Konnerth CG & Hummel T (2004). A study on the frequency of olfactory dysfunction. *Laryngoscope,* 114(10):1764-9

Levine HL (1990). Functional endoscopic sinus surgery: evaluation, surgery and follow-up of 250 patients. *Laryngoscope,* 100:79-84

Lildholdt T (1989). Surgical versus medical treatment of nasal polyps. *Rhinol Suppl,* 8:31-33

Lildholdt T, Rundcrantz H & Lindqvist N (1995). Efficacy of corticosteroid powder for nasal polyps: a double-blind, placebo-controlled study of budesonide. *Clin Otolaryngol Allied Sci,* 20:26-30

Litvack JR, Fong K, Mace J, James KE & Smith TL (2008). Predictors of olfactory dysfunction in patients with chronic rhinosinusitis. *Laryngoscope,* 118(12): 2225-2230

Litvack JR, Mace J & Smith TL (2009b). Does olfactory function improve after endoscopic sinus surgery? *Otolaryngol Head Neck Surg,* 140:312-319

Litvack JR, Mace JC & Smith TL (2009a). Olfactory function and disease severity in chronic rhinosinusitis. *Am J Rhinol Allergy,* 23(2):139-144

Lund VJ & MacKay IS (1994). Outcome assessment of endoscopic sinus surgery. *J R Soc Med,* 87:70-72

Lund VJ & Scadding GK (1994). Objective assessment of sinus surgery in the management of chronis rhinosinusitis: an update. *J Laryngol Otol,* 108:749-753

Min YG, Yun YS, Song BH, Cho YS & Lee KS (1995). Recovery of nasal physiology after functional endoscopic sinus surgery: olfaction and mucociliary transport. *ORL J Otorhinolaryngol Relat Spec,* 57:264-268

Miwa T, Furukawa M, Tsukatani T, Costanzo RM, DiNardo LJ & Reiter ER (2001). Impact of olfactory impairment on quality of life and disability. *Arch Otolaryngol Head Neck Surg,* 127(5):497-503

Mott AE & Leopold DA (1991). Disorders in taste and smell. *Med Clin North Am,* 75:1321-1353

Mott AE, Cain WS, Lafreniere D, Leonard G, Gent JF & Frank ME (1997). Topical corticosteroid treatment of anosmia associated with nasal and sinus disease. *Arch Otolaryngol Head Neck Surg,* 123:367-372

Murphy C, Shubert CR, Cruickshanks KJ, Klein BE, Klein R & Nondahl DM (2002). Prevalence of olfactory impairment in older adults. *JAMA,* 288:2307-2312

Mygind N, Nielsen LP, Hoffmann HJ, Shukla A, Blumberga G, Dahl R & Jacobi H (2001) Mode of action of intranasal corticosteroids. *J Allergy Clin Immunol,* 108 (1Suppl):S16-25

Naessen R (1971). An inquiry on the morphological characteristics and possible changes with age in the olfactory regions of man. *Acta Otolaryngol,* 71:49-62

Nakashima T, Kimmelman C & Snow JB (1985). Immunohistopathology of human olfactory nerve epithelium, nerve and bulb. *Laryngoscope,* 95:391-398

Neuland C, Bitter T, Marschner H, Gudziol H & Gutinas-Lichius O (2011). Health-related and specific olfaction-related quality of life in patients with chronic functional anosmia or severe hyposmia. *Laryngoscope,* 121(4):867:72

Nordin S, Monsch AU & Murphy C (1995). Unawareness of smell loss in normal aging and Alzheimer's disease: discrepancy between self-reported and diagnosed smell sensitivity. *J Gerontol B Psychol Sci Soc Sci,* 50(4):187-82

Orlandi RR & Terrell JE (2002). Analysis of the adult chronic rhinosinusitis working definition. *Am J Rhinol,* 16:7-10

Park AH, Lau J, Stankiewicz J & Chow J (1998). The role of functional endoscopic sinus surgery in asthmatic patients. *J Otolaryngol,* 27:275-280

Raviv JR & Kern KC (2004). Chronic rhinosinusitis and olfactory dysfunction. *Otolaryngol Clin North Am,* 37:1143-1157

Reden J, Maroldt H, Fritz A, Zahnert T & Hummel T (2007). A study on the prognostic significance of qualitative olfactory dysfunction. *Eur Arch Otorhinolaryngol,* 264(2):139-44

Rombaux P, Mouraux A, Bertrand B, Guerit JM & Hummel T (2006). Assessment of olfactory and trigeminal function using chemosensory event-related potentials. *Neurophysiol Clin,* 36(2):53-62

Rombaux P, Mouraux A, Collet S, Eloy P & Bertrand B (2009). Usefulness and feasibility of psychophysical and electrophysiological olfactory testing in rhinology clinic. *Rhinology,* 47(1):28-35

Rombaux P,Potier H, Bertrand B, Duprez T & Hummel T (2008). Olfactory bulb volume in patients with sinonasal disease. *Am J Rhinol,* 22(6):598-601

Seiden AM & Duncan HJ (2001). The diagnosis of conductive olfactory loss. *Laryngoscope,* 111:9-14

Simola M & Malmberg H (1998). Sense of smell in allergic and non-allergic rhinitis. *Allergy,* 53:190-194

Soler ZM, Mace J & Smith TL (2008). Symptom-based presentation of chronic rhinosinusitis before and after functional endoscopic sinus surgery. *Am J Rhinol,* 22:297-301

Soler ZM, Sauer DA, Mace JC & Smith TL (2010). Ethmoid histopathology does not predict olfactory outcomes after endoscopic sinus surgery. *Am J Rhinol Allergy,* 24(4):281-5

Stuck BA, Blum A, Hagner AE, Hummel T, Klimek L & Hörmann K (2003). Mometasone furoate nasal spray improves olfactory performances in seasonal allergic rhinitis. *Allergy,* 58:1195

Temmel AF, Quint C, Schickinger-Fischer B, Klimek L, Stoller E & Hummel T (2002). Characteristics of olfactory disorders in relation to major causes of olfactory loss. *Arch Otolaryngol Head Neck Surg,* 128:635-641

Tourbier IA & Doty RL (2007). Sniff magnitude test: relationship to odor identification, detection and memory tests in a clinic population. *Chem Sens,* 32(6):515-23

Vaidyanathan S, Barnes M, Williamson P, Hopkinson P, Donnan PT & Lipworth B (2011). Treatment of chronic rhinosinusitis with nasal polyposis with oral steroids followed by topical steroids: and randomized trial. *An Intern Med,* 154(5):293:302

Vento SI, Simola M, Ertama LO & Malmberg CHO (2001). Sense of smell in longstanding nasal polyposis. *Am J Rhinol,* 15:159-163

Wang JH, Kwon HJ & Jang YJ (2010). Staphylococcus aureus increases cytokine and matrix metalloproteinase expression in nasal mucosa of patients with chronic rhinosinusitis and nasal polyps. *Am J Rhinol Allergy,* 24(6):422-7

Welge-Luessen A (2009). Psychophysical effects of nasal and oral inflammation. *Ann N Y Acad Sci,* 1170:585-9

Wright ED & Agrawal S (2007). Impact of perioperative systemic steroids on surgical outcomes in patients with chronic rhinosinusitis with polyposis: evaluation with novel perioperative sinus endoscopy (POSE) scoring system. *Laryngoscope,* 117 (11 Pt 2 Suppl 115): 1-28

Yee KK, Pribitkin EA, Cowart BJ, Vainius AA, Klock CT, Rosen D, Feng P, Mc Lean J, Hahn CG & Rawson NE (2010). Neuropathology of the olfactory mucosa in chronic rhinosinusitis. *Am J Rhinol Allergy,* 24(2):110-20

4

Refractory Chronic Rhinosinusitis: Etiology & Management

Mohannad Al-Qudah
Jordan University of Science & Technology,Irbid, Jordan

1. Introduction

Chronic rhinosinusitis (CRS) is a common disease with significant morbidity and health care cost. Although the medical and surgical treatments for CRS have improved markedly over the past few decades, a subset of patients remains quite resistant to all forms of therapy.

Such patients end up being over-treated and subjected to numerous unsuccessful surgeries some of which can result in serious complications. The optimal treatment for these patients (an entity referred to as refractory or recalcitrant sinusitis) (RCRS) is complex and challenging.

The true incidenceof RCRS is unknown. It is estimated that at least 10 % of patients with CRS continue to be symptomatic after appropriate endoscopic sinus surgery (ESS) with long term follow up. This 10% failure rate translates into 30,000 patients yearlyundergoing ESS with poor postoperative outcome.Because these numbers are cumulative over years, approximately450,000 cases in the United States are currently estimatedto have chronic sinusitis that is unresponsive to medical and surgical therapy. Today, these chronic patients form a significant portion of most rhinology practices. (Desrosiers, 2004).

The aims of this chapter are to review the updated possible pathogesis of RCRS and suggest possible algorithmic management plan for this condition.

2. History and physical examinations

Thoroughand detailed history is fundamental in evaluating patients to find out whether optimal treatment has been given, and whether there are any personal or technical predisposing factors.

Current symptomatology should be determined. Detailed questions regarding nasal symptoms: facial pressure, nasal obstruction, anterior or posterior rhinorrhea,and alteration of sense of smell should be asked. Frequency and duration of symptoms exacerbation as well as different modalities of treatments used should be reviewed.

Routine medical questions should also be included. Specific attention should be paid to thesymptoms of respiratory system, such as cough, wheeze, and shortness of breath.History of recurrent infections in the skin, urinary tract or digestive tract may indicate immunodeficiency. Additionally, connective tissue disorders, granulomatous diseases and vasculatitis related symptoms need be asked.

Medication should be reviewed and the use of oral immunosuppressive agents determined.

Allergy questionnaires should cover presence of household pets or excess mold in the domestic environment. Work history should be obtained to evaluate occupational causative elements to the disease. Both smoking historyand passive exposure to smoke should be assessed.

Previous nasal surgeries reviewed. Type of surgery, recovery, complications and response should all be documented.

Complete ear, nose, and throat examination is followed. Anterior rhinoscopy should assess nasal patency, nasal mucosa condition, inferior turbinates, and the presence of nasal crusting.

Direct visualization using 0 and 30 degree rigid endoscopy is crucial in this group of patients, to look for any evidenceof active infection or obstruction to sinus ostium. The presence of polyps, pus,synechiae,stenosis, middle turbinate lateralization should also be evaluated.Pathological looking mucosa can be biopsied under local anesthesia as office procedure to rule out systemic diseases or tumors.

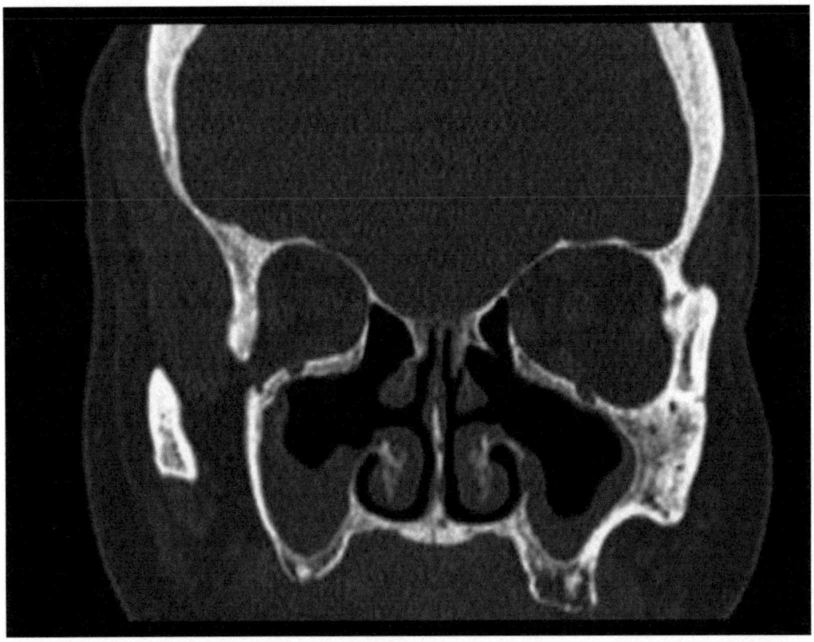

Fig. 1. Coronal CT scan for patient with RCRS, thickened mucosa with patent sinus ostium and Osteitis of the left lateral maxillary wall.

If surgery is not technically adequate and evidence of obstruction noticed revision surgery is offered.

Thin cut CT scan with coronal and sagital reconstruction should be ordered. CT scan can illustrate detail in lateral wall of sinuses where the endoscopic view cannot reach.Extent of sinus involvement, extent of prior surgery, presence of obstruction to sinus drainage, unventilated cells, development of new bone deposition or neo-osteogenesis, and evidence of previous intraoperative complications can be easily visualized. Figure 1 showed the typical CT scan finding in patients with RCRS.

3. Pathogenesis and treatment

3.1 Immunodeficiency & RCRS

Although the exact role of bacteria and fungus in the etiology of sinusitis is still controversial, we have reasonable evidences to believe they play significant role in this wide spectrum disease. Bacteria and fungus have been detected in endoscopic guided culture, type of organisms identified in acute sinusitis differs from those reported in chronic and in RCRS. In general, patients with sinusitis report improvement in their symptoms while they are on Antibiotics. Additionally, the prevalence &severity of sinusitis in immuncompromised patients correlate with their immunological status. In fact, Antimicrobial therapy is still the mostcommon form of therapy prescribed by physiciansfor the treatment of CRS.

Various forms of immunodeficiencies predispose to rhinosinusitis, however in RCRS the most important are selective IgA deficiency and systemic subtle humoral immunodeficiencies. These patients are usually diagnosed after being treated with multiple sinus surgeries. Other forms of immunodeficiency, for example, common variable immunodeficiency lymphopenia or neutropenia are more important in the pathogenesis of recurrent acute forms of rhinosinusitis and acute invasive fungal sinusitis.

Immune dysfunction as a risk factor for RCRS has gained attention in recent years.Chee et al studied the incidence of primary immune deficiency in patients with refractory sinusitis.Among a group of 79 patients with refractory sinusitis 17.9% were noted to have low IgG and 16.7% were noted to have low IgA. Common variable immunodeficiency was found in 9.9% and selective IgA deficiency was diagnosed in 6.2%. Although these numbers are interesting, the authors included some patients who didn't fit with the current definition of RCRS, they defined refractory sinusitis as at least one previous sinussurgery and/or three episodes of objectively documented rhinosinusitis in the previous year (Cheel et al., 2001).

Vanleberghe et al. reported on a series of cases with RCRS whohad undergone immunologic evaluation. Out of 307(261 adults and 46 children) patients tested, 22% had evidence of humoral immunodeficiency.The majority of these were subtle IgG subclass deficits, low level of major immunoglobulins was reported in 7% for IgA and 3.3%.for IgG. Low level of IgM or Common variable immunodeficiency weren't detected (Vanlerberghe et al., 2006).

In a recent paper Al-Qudah et al studied the contribution of primary immunodeficiency in 67 patients with RCRS at a large tertiary care medical center. In addition to major immunoglobulin and IgG subclasses blood level, Functional antibody response was assessed by examining the antibody response to the unconjugated pneumococcal polysaccharide vaccine. Low IgG was detected in 9%, low IgA in 3%, low IgM in 12% of patients, and IgG subclasses in 19%. Common variable immunodeficiency was diagnosed in one case. 67% of patients failed to produce more than a fourfold increase in postimmunization antibody titer for 7 of 14 serotypes being tested and were considered to have functional antibody deficiency. Interestingly there was no statistically significant difference in the incidence of low level of immunoglobulins between patients with normal antibody response and poor response group. They recommended measurement of serumimmunoglobulin levels in all patients with RCRS; if these are normal, then functional antibody responses should be evaluated (Alqudah et al., 2010).

Functional antibody responses or selective antibody deficiency syndrome is a condition with normal or near normal serum immunoglobulin concentrations but an inadequate production of specific antibodies response to polysaccharide organisms, which are T-independent type 2 antigens, like Streptococcus pneumonia. Patient with this condition have recurrent respiratory infections such as: sinusitis, bronchitis, and pneumonia.The diagnosis can be reached by taking paired blood sample before and 6-weks after immunization with pneumococcal vaccine.The consensus recommendation is that a normal response in adultsis a fourfold increase in antibody titers to 70% of the14 serotypesunconjugated pneumococcal polysaccharide and a normal response in children is a fourfold increase in antibody titers to 50% of the serotypes tested (Bonilla et al.,2005).

T cell immunodeficiency patients are unlikely to present with Refractory sinusitis symptoms without other apparent clinical presentation. Primary T cell disorders are rare and usually diagnosed during childhood. Secondary T cell deficiency presents with unusual or severe viral, fungal or protozoal infection.

Food allergy is another possible cause of persistent nasal symptoms after proper medical and surgical therapy especially in patient with nasal polyp. Most common "masked" food allergens in adults are those foods commonly eaten and include: wheat, dairy, soy, corn, and, eggs (Ferguson et al., 2009).

The condition is usually difficult to recognize by the patients as symptoms may show up hours or even a day after food absorption and the fact that common allergic foods are so prevalent in our diet that many patients eat them nearly every day. An elimination food challenging test is a convenient and inexpensive procedure that can performed by the patient at home. The targeted food is eliminated from the diet for 5 to 7 days and then reintroduced into the diet during this hyperresponsive period of 5 to 10 days following elimination. If the food causes symptoms, then the patient will generally be aware of either nasal or non-nasal symptoms after the food challenge. Those who note symptoms on reintroduction of the food are instructed to eliminate the food from their diet for approximately 3 months, after which time the food may be reintroduced into their diet, although the food should not be eaten on a daily basis (Ozdemir et al., 2009).

Our immune evaluation for patients with RCRS is displayed in Table 1.All patients should have complete blood cell count with differential, measurement of serum IgG, IgA, IgM, IgE and IgG subclasses as well as allergy skin test or radioallergosorbent test. If serum immunoglobulin levels are normal, functional antibody responses should be evaluated by determining specific antibody response to an unconjugated pneumococcal polysaccharide vaccine.

Complete blood cell count with differential
Quantitative immunoglobulins: IgA, IgE, IgM, IgG and IgG subclasses
Allergy Test.
Pneumococcal antibody titers

Table 1. Immune work up in refractory chronic sinusitis

In addition to twice daily nasal irrigations and long term nasal steroid all RCRS patients with immunodeficiency need to be on prophylactic oral antibiotics. Our protocol is to use two different antibiotics rotating every two weeks and so any emerging resistant clones will wipe out with the other antibiotic. For many reasons, Bactrim and Doxycycline are our first option: They are old, cheap, safe antibiotics and prescribed twice daily. Additionally these two antibiotics have a potent anti-inflammatory effect. Cephalexin, Amoxcillin and Clarithromycin are alternative options for those patients who are allergic or can't tolerate Bactrim and Doxycycline. The duration of prophylactic antibiotics use is flexible and depends mainly on patient's symptoms duration and clinical response. Antibiotics can be used all through the year or given in symptomatic season. Acute exacerbation is treated according to endoscopic guided culture. Patients who failed to improve on antibiotics can benefit from intravenous or subcutaneous immunoglobulin replacement. The recommended stander dose is 400-600 mg/kg given every four weeks for 1-2 years. (Shearer et al 1996).

Cessation of treatment is schedule during summer months to avoid allergy season and to avoid the high incidence of infections during winter.

3.2 Biofilm & RCRS

Biofilms are a complex organized community of germs that adhere to the mucosal surface and surrounded by a self-produced extensive extracellular polymeric substance called (glycocalyx) which composed primarily of polysaccharides. The glycocalyx is a mixture of bacterial colonies of different phenotypes with various physiochemical properties. It serves as protection for its bacterial inhabitants while also modulating the microenvironment of the colonies through its numerous water channels. Biofilms intermittently release free floating bacteria (planktonic) that can provide a constant nidus of infection.

Biofilm's life cycle and interactions with the environment can be divided into three stages: attachment, growth, and detachment. During the attachment phase,the substratum has to be adequate for the reversible adsorption and ultimately the irreversible attachment of bacteria to the surface. During the growth phase, as thecells divide and colonize the surface, a polysaccharide matrix is formed, and the biofilm begins to display athree-dimensional structure. During this phase water channels are formed. Once biofilms reach maturity, bacteria slough off and embolize to other areaswhere the process may begin again (Sanclement et al.,2005).

Bacterial biofilms have two microbiological characteristic: first, they are difficult to detect and culture using routine conventional methods and second, they are 10-1000 time resistant to current antimicrobial therapy when compared with genetically identical planktonic bacteria (Kilty & Desrosiers, 2009).

Antibiotics resistance is most likely related to biofilm slow growth and metabolic rate as well as sharing of multiple resistance genes within the members of the biofilm community. Antibiotic treatment will kill bacteria in the periphery where the cells are metabolically active, but doesn't reach the bacteria in the deeper layers of the biofilm. Thus, the biofilm serves as a bacterial reservoir that sheds planktonic forms causing systemic illness, especially when released intothe circulation. In these circumstances, antibiotic treatment will eliminate the circulating bacteria but not the biofilm, leading to recurring acute exacerbations (Post et al., 2007).

Biofilm infection theory may offer an explanation of the high rate of negative sinus cavities in CRS and why antibiotic treatment is unable to resolve CRS with bacteria that are sensitive to antibiotics.In 2004, Cryer and his colleagues were first to demonstrate the presence of biofilms in the biopsied mucosa from a number of symptomatic CRS patients who had prior appropriate medical and surgical management (Cryer et al.,2004) .One year later Ramadan et al identified biofilms on the mucosa of five patients at the time of ESS.(Ramadan,2006).

Further studies found significant differences in the rate of biofilms formation between control, CRS and refractory sinusitis (Bendouah et al., 2006; Psaltis et al., 2007; Sanclement et al., 2005).

Another support to the biofilm theory is that pathogenic bacteria most commonly implicated in RCRS have been identified in patients with RCRS to exist in the form of a biofilm. In several studies of bacteriology in RCRS performed with conventional culture methods, Staphylococcus aureus, Coagulase negative staphylococci and Pseudomonas aeruginosa have been identified as the most common bacteria to colonize the paranasal sinuses and these same species were the most common bacteria identified in the biofilms of refractory sinusitis patients using different invasive labartory techniques.

The preoperative presence and type of bacteria biofims in sinus mucosa may correlate with continuous postoperative symptoms and mucosal inflammation after ESS. Bendouahet et al took 31 isolates from 19 CRS patients who had undergone ESS a year earlier. 71% of isolates showed biofilm formation. Among the bacteria recovered, Pseudomonas aeruginosa and Staphylococcus aureus biofilm was shown to have a correlation with poor outcome after ESS, whereas Coagulase negative staphylococci biofilm did not (Bendouah et al., 2006). More recently, Psaltis et al retrospectively studied a group of 40 CRS patients who had undergone ESS. Outcome measures revealed that bacterial biofilms were found in 50 percent of the 40 patients and that the poorer post operation symptoms were correlated with the presence of bacterial biofilms. Interestingly biofims formation is independent of many common risk factors,(such as allergy, polyps, samter's triad) cited in the etiology of CRS were not found to be of significant in (Psaltis et al., 2008).

Staphylococcus aureus, Pseudomonas aeruginosa and Coagulase negative staph. are the most frequent biofilm forming bacteria in RCRS, these bacteria are usually resistant to oral and intravenous antibiotics at minimum inhibitory concentration (MIC). In a study aimed to determine the in vitro activity of moxifloxacin against Staphylococcus aureus in biofilm form with samples recovered from patients with at least 1 year post-ESS, the authors found moxifloxacin at 1000 times the known MIC was statistically significant in reducing the number of viable bacteria (Desrosiers et al., 2007).

In another work, authors studied the MIC of different antibiotics to eradicate Pseudomonas aeruginosa biofilms, they found The minimum biofilm eradication concentration for

Pseudomonas biofilms has been shown to be 60-fold greater than the MIC for gentamicin and greater than 1000-fold for ceftazidime and piperacillin(Ceri, 1999)

These date and others encourage rhinologist in the past few years toward treating Biofilms in RCRS with different delivery methods of topical antibiotics at concentration above the MIC level with minimum systemic side effects, taking advantage of the anatomical and physiological changes after ESS where paranasal sinuses become single large cavity connected with multiple patent ostiums.

Antibiotics can deliver into nasal cavity by nasal sprays, irrigations, nebulizers or by direct installation using syringe and large gauge needle. Because nasal sprays rely on mucociliary clearance to transport the drug, and this is often impaired in RCRS, as well as their small surface area deposition many believe this method of delivery is suboptimum(Lim et al, 2008,Richard et al ,2010).

Most of clinical research on topical antibiotics for RCRS is limited with small number of patients, short follow up, different protocols for treatment and inclusions and exclusions criteria, however The conclusion of 2 recent review articles support the use of topical antibiotics in RCRS and recommend the need of larger and better designed randomized double-blinded placebo-controlled studies (Lim et al, 2008,Richard et al ,2010)

3.3 Osteitis and neo-osteogenesis in RCRS

Although CRS begins in the mucosa there are evidences that inflammation can spread and involve underlying bony structures leading to persistent of patients' symptoms following aggressive medical and proper surgical treatment.The mucosa and underlying bone are not separated units and they wee communicate with each other.

Bolger et al studied the histopathology changes after induce sinus infection in 33 New Zealand white rabbits with Pseudomonas aeruginosa. Histologic analysis of the bone 4, 14, 21, and 28 days after bacterial infection showed stromal changes of bone resorption, reactive osteoblasts, and appositional or intra-membranous new bone formation as early as 4 days after bacterial inoculation. Bacteria were present in the sinus lumen, surface of sinus mucosa, mucosal crypts, mucosal abscesses, and ulcers but not in the bone itself. They conclude that although bacteria were limited to the mucosa, the infection induced histopathological changes at the submucosa and bone level (Bolger et al., 1997). Using the same model and pathogen, Perloff and colleagues confirmed these bony changes to be identical to chronic osteomyelitis, interestingly, in all studied specimens some bony changes were found at the non-infected side . They suggested that inflammation may travel along bone to adjacent sinuses without intervening mucosal disease. Properly inflammatory or infectious agents entered the underlying bone, through Haversian canals, and subsequently activated the remodeling process in sites distant or adjacent to the original inoculation site (Perloff et al.,2000).

In another study, 14 rabbits were induced by Staphylococcus aureus, chronic osteomyelitis in the non-infected side was found in (43%) (Khalid et al., 2002).

Bony changes had been also reported in studies on patients with CRS.Kennedy et al noted marked activity with features of increased fibrosis, remodeling, and woven bone in ethmoid labyrinth. Ethmoid septations were found to have evidence of marked acceleration in bone physiology with histologic findings including presence of inflammatory cells, fibrosis, and new bone formation. They also reported inflammation in the bone even when the overlying mucosa was intact (Kennedy, 1998).

Giacchiet al. compared bone from ethmoid septa of 20 patients with CRS and control group.Those with CRS typically showed periosteal thickening and resorption or remodeling. They also found a trend toward more advanced histologic bone stage associated with higher CT score indicating that mucosal and bone pathological changes occurred simultaneously (Giacchi et al.,2001).

In a recent study from Netherland , the authors used CT scan to report the incidence of osteitis in 102 CRS patients and in an age- and gender matched control group of 68 non-CRS patients. Forty per cent of the CRS group and none of the control group had evidence of clinically significant osteitis. In the CRS group the severity of osteitis was correlated with Lund–Mackay score ($P < 0.001$), duration of symptoms ($P < 0.01$) and previous surgery ($P < 0.001$). The association between osteitis and number of previous surgery remained strong even after adjusting for the disease duration. There was no association between osteitis and age, gender, smoking, co-existing asthma, allergy or Sumter's triad (Georgalas et al. 2010)

Osteitis and neo-osteogenesis may also affect the success rate after sinus surgery. Kim et al studied the correlation between pre-operative bony changes detected in CT scan and postoperative endoscopic signs of healed sinus cavities in 81 patients. Patients with no radiological signs of bony changes showed better healing mucosa compare to those with bony changes (Kim et al., 2006).

Pathological changes described by human histological studies included: the presence of new bone formation, fibrosis, inflammatory cells, periosteal thickening and a varying degree of increased osteoblastic- osteoclastic activity, as shown by the disruption of organised lamellar bone and formation of immature woven bone, these are best to fit under the terms ostitis and neo-osteogesis. Localized or generalized thickened, irregular, heterogeneous lining of the sinus walls, is the radiological sign observed in CT scan, as illustrated in Figure 2 (Georgalas et al., 2010).

Osteitis and neo-osteogenesisin CRS are probably secondary to inflammatory process rather than direct bacterial invasion. In all animals and human studies, bacteria were not detected in the inflamed bone except in Tovi's study where actinomycosis was found in one patient (Tovi et al., 1992).

Cytokines produced by inflammatory cells such as osteoclast activating factor, interleukins, and tumor necrosis factor as well as prostaglandins such as prostaglandin 2 are known stimulators of bone resorption. These could be important mediators in inflammatory bone resorption and bone loss such as in periodontal disease and arthritis(9). Prostaglandin E is also shown to cause hyperostosis with periosteal osteoblast proliferation, thickened periosteum, and neocortex formation (Kocak et al., 2002; Faye-Petersen et al., 1996).

Mechanical pressure resulting from increased intrasinus pressure caused by inflammation and ostiomeatal unit obstruction may stimulate bone remodeling. This could explain the trend toward more advanced bone stage associated with higher CT stage of mucosal disease observed by Giacchi et al .

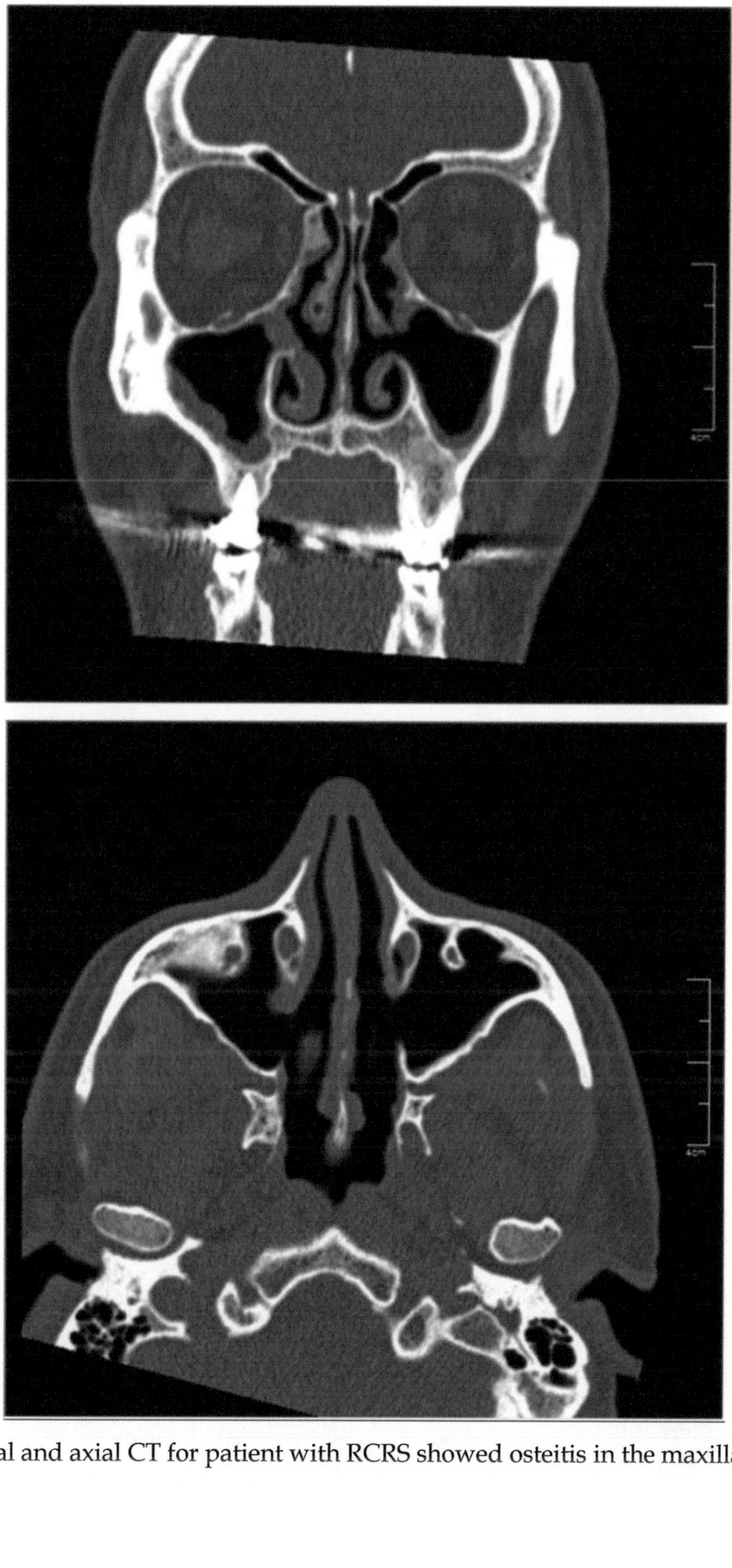

Fig. 2. Coronal and axial CT for patient with RCRS showed osteitis in the maxillary wall.

Another possible explanation is bacterial Biofilms may act as a 'depot' for low grade bacterial production and be responsible for the release of soluble bacterial virulence factors that generate local bony changes. The authors of most studies on biofilms and sinusitis didn't specify whether their sinus samples where purely mucosal or with some bony fragments, biofilms have been reported to present in infected bone in orthopedic and dental literature. Indeed, further studies are needed to determine the exact role of biolms in osteitis in RCRS.

Long therapeutic plan required in management of these patients. Complete removal of crust and sequestered bone is essential first step to provide healthy environment for mucosal regeneration. Topical combination of antibiotic and steroid may also help.

3.4 Granulomatous disease and vasculitis in RCRS

The sinonasal cavity may be the first organ to manifest such a systemic condition. Presenting symptoms and signs may be identical to those of other forms of CRS and thus these patients may have delay diagnosis.

The list of granulomatous diseases that can affect the sinonasal tract is extensive Sarcoidosis, Wegener's granulomatosis, Churg- Strauss syndrome, are the most common. Detailed history, carful systemic examination and local biopsy of any abnormal looking mucosa may be the hint of early identification of these patients.

Sarcoidosis is an inflammatory multisystem disorder of characterized by noncaseating granulomas. Sinonasal cavity is affected in only 0.7% to 6% of cases. Symptoms that may point to sarcoidosis are fatigue, pulmonary symptoms, night sweating, weight loss and fever.Physicalsigns include mucosal hypertrophy, purple mucosa with nodules (granulomas), and lupus pernio. Diagnosis is based on clinical findings, chest radiography, elevated angiotensin-converting enzyme levels, and findings of mucosal biopsy from affected mucosa (Matthew, 2008; Ferguson et al., 2009).

Wegener's granulomatosis is a rare granulomatous vasculitic disorder, affecting primarilymiddle age white people.Sinonasal manifestations are very common and occur in up to 89% of patients.Common symptoms include nasal obstruction, bloody rhinorrhea, epiphora, and crusting. Patients may present with, septal perforation, mucocele, orbital pseudotumor, or saddle-nose deformity. Positive cytoplasmic antineutrophil cytoplasmic antibodies and an elevated erythrocyte sedimentation rate suggest the diagnosis. However, definitive diagnosis depends on histopathologic analysis of affected mucosa.

Churg–Strauss syndrome is a multisystem disorder with necrotizing granulomatous eosinophilic tissue infiltration. Nasal involvement can occur in up to 75% of patients. Nasal polyps and rhinosinusitis are early manifestations of the illness, with subsequent development of eosinophilia and systemic involvement. Diagnosis is based on clinical findings, positive perinuclearantineutrophil cytoplasmic antibodies, and biopsy.

Treatment of nasal granulomatous diseases most commonly includes aggressive sinus debridement to remove crust formation, saline rinses and topical, systemic, intralesional steroids and immunosuppressive medications, surgery is reserved for complicated cases. Early consultation with rheumatology and immunology teams is essential for proper management plan(Ryan 2008, Ferguson and Otto 2009).

3.5 Gastroesophageal reflux disease

Gastroesophageal reflux disease (GERD) has been implicated as a contributing factor in many air way disease processes like: dysphonia, benign vocal cord lesions, vocal laryngospasm, subglottic stenosis, asthma, CRS, post nasal drip and idiopathic cough.

Three mechanisms could explain the effect of GERD on sinusitis: direct exposure of the nasopharynx and nose to gastric acid causing mucosal inflammation and impaired mucociliary clearance, the second possible mechanism is a dysfunction of the autonomous nervous system resulting in vagus nerve stimulation, the third possible mechanism relates to the direct role of Helicobacter pylori.

DelGaudio was first to document nasopharyngeal reflux (NPR) in RCRS patients, in prospective study using 24 hour pH study with a specially designed probe with sensors located in the nasopharynx, 1 cm above the upper esophageal sphincter, and the distal esophagus.

He found significant differences in the number of patients with NPR events (pH less than 5) and GERD between patients with RCRS and two control groups, the first consisted of patients who had at least one ESS procedure and had no symptoms of CRS or mucosal inflammation with a minimum of 1 year postoperative follow up. The second control group consisted of subjects with no history of CRS or sinus surgery. Limitation of this paper was that the study and control groups were not matched for age and comorbidities. The study group was older than the control group by approximately 10 years, and also, the study group patientshave more comorbid conditions, especially asthma, comparedwith the control group. This weakness may question the accuracy of the results and conclusions (DelGaudio, 2005).

In prospective study, DiBaise et al treated 11 RCRS patients with proton pump inhibitor, not all patients had frank symptoms of GERD, Individual sinus symptoms (nasal congestion, nasal drainage, sinus pressure, facial headache, malaise) and global satisfaction were modestly improved in 25-89% and 91%, respectively, at 12 week (DiBaise et al.,2002).

Flook and Kumar conducted a recent review analysis for the evidence to link acid reflux with chronic sinusitis or any nasal symptoms; their conclusion was that the evidence of a link is poor with no good randomized controlled trials available. The few adult studies that show any link between acid reflux and nasal symptoms are small case-controlled studies with moderate levels of potential bias. There is not enough evidence to consider anti-reflux therapy for adult refractory CRS and there is no evidence that acid reflux is a significant causal factor in CRS (Flook & Kumar, 2011).

In our practice, we don't referred asymptomatic patients with RCRS for 24-hour Ph monitoring; however we started all RCRS patients on 20mg omeprazole BID for 3 weeks, if patient reports improvement in nasal symptoms or endoscopic score we recommend to continue on this regimen for 12 weeks.

4. Conclusions

A group of CRS patients continue to be symptomatic after appropriate medical and surgical therapy. Detailed history, endoscopic examination, laboratory and immunology tests required to look for any reversible underlying pathology. Further clinical studies and in vitro research are in great needed to support and validate the current management protocol. The current treatment of RCRS is by nasal toilet, debridement, prophylactic antibiotics and immunoglobulin as well as topical medications.

5. References

Alqudah M, Graham SM, BallasZK. *High prevalence of humoral immunodeficiency patients with refractory chronic rhinosinusitis.*Am J Rhinol Allergy. 2010 Nov;24(6):409-12.

Bonilla FA, Bernstein IL, Khan DA, Ballas ZK, Chinen J, Frank MM, Kobrynski LJ, Levinson AI, Mazer B, Nelson RP Jr, Orange JS, Routes JM, Shearer WT, Sorensen RU.(2005). *Practice parameter for the diagnosis and management of primary immunodeficiency.*Ann Allergy Asthma Immunol. ,Vol.94,No.5 Suppl 1,pp.S1-63

Bendouah Z, Barbeau J, Hamad WA, et al.(2006). Biofilm formation by Staphylococcus aureus and Pseudomonas aeruginosa is associated with an unfavorable evolution after surgery for chronic sinusitis and nasal polyposis. Otolaryngol Head Neck Surg,Vol.134,No.6,pp.991–6.

Bolger W, Leonard D, Dick E, et al.(1997).Gram negative sinusitis: a bacteriologic and histologic study in rabbits. Am J Rhinol, Vol.11,pp.15–25.

Ceri H, Olson ME, Stremick C, et a (1999)l.: The Calgary Biofilm Device: new technology for rapid determination of antibiotic susceptibilities of bacterial biofilms. J Clin Microbiol ,37:1771–1776.

Chee L, Graham SM, Carothers DG, Ballas ZK.(2001). *Immune dysfunction in refractory sinusitis in a tertiary care setting.* Laryngoscope, Vol.111,pp.233–235.

Cryer J, Schipor I, Perloff JR, Palmer JN.(2004).Evidence of bacterial biofilms in human chronic sinusitis.*ORL J OtorhinolaryngolRelat Spec.* Vol.66,No.3,pp.155-8.

DesrosiersM.(2004).*Refractory chronic rhinosinusitis: pathophysiology and management of chronic rhinosinusitis persisting after endoscopic sinus surgery.*Curr Allergy Asthma Rep, Vol4,No.3,pp.200-7.

Desrosiers M, Bendouah Z, Barbeau J(2007): Effectiveness of topical antibiotics on Staphylococcus aureus biofilm in vitro. Am J Rhinol ,Vol 21:149–153.

DelGaudioJM(2005). *Direct nasopharyngeal reflux of gastric acid is a contributing factor in refractory chronic rhinosinusitis.* Laryngoscope.Vol.115,No.6,pp.946-57.

DiBaise JK, Olusola BF, Huerter JV, Quigley EM(2002).Role of GERD in chronic resistant sinusitis: a prospective, open label, pilot trial.*Am J Gastroenterol.*Vol.97,No.4,pp.843-50.

Ferguson BJ, Otto BA, Pant H.(2009).*When surgery, antibiotics, and steroids fail to resolve chronic rhinosinusitis.*Immunol Allergy Clin North Am.Vol29,No.4,pp.719-32

Flook EP, Kumar BN.(2011).Is there evidence to link acid reflux with chronic sinusitis or any nasal symptoms? A review of the evidence.*Rhinology.*Vol.49,No.1,pp.11-6.

Faye-Petersen O, Johnson W, Carlo W, et al. Prostaglandin E1–induced hyperostosis: clinicopathologic correlations and possible pathogenic mechanisms. Ped Path Lab Med 1996, Vol.16,pp.489–507.

Ferguson BJ, Otto BA, Pant H.(2009).When surgery, antibiotics, and steroids fail to resolve chronic rhinosinusitis. *Immunol Allergy Clin North Am.*Vol,29,No.4,pp.719-32.

Giacchi R, Lebowitz R, Yee H, et al.(2001). *Histopathologic evaluation of the ethmoid bone in chronic sinusitis.* Am J Rhinol.Vol.15,pp.193–197.

Georgalas C.,* Videler W.,†Freling N. &Fokkens W.(2010). *Global Osteitis Scoring Scale and chronic rhinosinusitis: a marker of revision surgery.**

Georgalas C.,* Videler W.,†Freling N. &Fokkens W.**Global Osteitis Scoring Scale and chronic rhinosinusitis:a marker of revision surgery. ClinOtolaryngol.* Vol.35, No.6,pp.455-61

Kilty SJ, DesrosiersMY.(2009). *Are Biofilms the Answer in the Pathophysiology and Treatment of Chronic Rhinosinusitis? Immunol Allergy Clin North Am.* Vol.29, No.4,pp.645-56.

Khalid AN, Hunt J, Perloff JR, Kennedy DW(2002). *The role of bone in chronic rhinosinusitis.* Laryngoscope.Vol112,No.11,pp.1951-7.

Kennedy D, Senior B, Gannon F, et al.(1998). *Histology and histomorphometry of ethmoid bone in chronic rhinosinusitis.* Laryngoscope.Vol.108,pp.502–507.

Kim HY, Dhong HJ, Lee HJ, Chung YJ, Yim YJ, Oh JW, Chung SK, Kim HJ.(2006). *Hyperostosis may affect prognosis after primary endoscopic sinus surgery for chronic rhinosinusitis.* Otolaryngology–Head and Neck Surgery. Vol.135,pp.94-99.

Kocak, M; Smith T, MPH†; Smith M(2002). *Bone involvement in CRS, Current Opinion in Otolaryngology & Head & Neck Surgery.*Vol.10,Issue 1 ,pp 49-52

Matthew W. Ryan(2008). *Diseases associated with chronic rhinosinusitis: what is the significance?, Current Opinion in Otolaryngology & Head and Neck Surgery,*Vol.16,pp.231–236

Ozdemir O, Mete E, Catal F, et al.(2009).*Food intolerances and eosinophilic esophagitis in childhood.* Dig Dis Sci.Vol.54,pp.8–14.

Post JC, Hiller NL, Nistico L, Stoodley P, Ehrlich GD.(2007).The role of biofilms in otolaryngologic infections: update 2007. *CurrOpinOtolaryngol Head Neck Surg.*Vol.15,No.5,pp.347-51.

Psaltis AJ, Ha KR, Beule AG, et al.(2007).*Confocal scanning laser microscopy evidence of biofilms in patients with chronic rhinosinusitis.* Laryngoscope. Vol.117, No.7,pp.1302–6.

Psaltis AJ, Ha KR, Wormald PJ, et al.(2008).*The effect of bacterial biofilmson post-sinus surgical outcome.* Am J Rhinol.Vol.22,pp.1- 6.

Perloff J, Gannon F, Bolger W, et al.(2000).*Bone involvement in sinusitis: an apparent pathway of spread of disease.* Laryngoscope.Vol.110,pp.2095–2099.

Shearer WT, Buckley RH, Engler RJ, Finn AF Jr, Fleisher TA, Freeman TM, Herrod HG 3rd, Levinson AI, Lopez M, Rich RR, Rosenfeld SI, Rosenwasser LJ.(1996).Practice parameters for the diagnosis and management of immunodeficiency. The Clinical and Laboratory Immunology Committee of the American Academy of Allergy, Asthma, and Immunology (CLIC-AAAAI)*Ann Allergy Asthma Immunol.* Vol.76,No.3,pp.282-94.

Sanclement JA, Webster P, Thomas J, Ramadan HH.(2005). Bacterial Biofilms in Surgical Specimens of Patients with Chronic Rhinosinusitis *Laryngoscope.* Vol.115,No.4, pp.578-82.

Ramadan HH.(2006).*Chronic rhinosinusitis and bacterial biofilms.*CurrOpinOtolaryngol Head Neck Surg.Vol.14,No.3,pp.183-6

Tovi F, Benharroch D, Gatot A, et al.(1992).Osteoblasticosteitis of the maxillary sinus. Laryngoscope.Vol.102,pp.426–430

Vanlerberghe L, Joniau S, Jorissen M.(2006).*The prevalence of humoral immunodeficiency in refractory rhinosinusitis: a retrospective analysis.* B-ENT.Vol.2,pp.161–166.

Part 2

Diagnosis and Treatment of Rhinosinusitis

5

Imaging Rhinosinusitis

Heidi Beate Eggesbø
Oslo University Hospital, Rikshospitalet
Norway

1. Introduction

Rhinosinusitis is classified as acute, recurrent and chronic. The acute form of rhinosinusitis should be diagnosed on symptoms and clinical findings, and imaging should not be necessary unless inflammatory complications are suspected. In recurrent and chronic rhinosinusitis, imaging is important in making a diagnose and planning the treatment. It is also important to look for inflammatory complications, and to discriminate "simple rhinosinusitis" from fungal infection and neoplasm (Rosenfeld, 2007). Paranasal sinus anatomy and pathology are difficult to interpret correct. Therefore, experienced radiologists as well as optimal imaging with respect to modality and method is mandatory.

2. Imaging modalities

Four imaging modalities have been used for imaging rhinosinusitis.

1. Computed tomography (CT) is the "gold standard" in imaging recurrent and chronic rhinosinusitis. CT is perfect for demonstrating the complex bony paranasal sinus anatomy with its variants as well as the localisation and extent of soft the tissue masses. Further, during functional endoscopic sinus surgery (FESS), the coronal or multiplanar CT is used as a bony map. Imaging rhinosinusitis without suspected complications, no intravenous contrast medium is needed (Eggesbo, 1999).
2. Magnetic resonance imaging (MRI) is complementary to CT, when CT has revealed soft tissue masses. In case of advanced unilateral soft tissue masses, MR imaging is mandatory to rule out, or further characterise fungal infection and neoplasm.
3. Plain films do not delineate the bony anatomy or soft tissue masses adequately and therefore this examination no longer have a place in imaging rhinosinusitis. The use of plain films should be limited to cases where CT is not available.
4. Ultrasonography has been used to detect pathology in the maxillary sinuses and anterior nasal fossa, however, the literature is not conclusive of its role in imaging rhinosinusitis.

The radiation dose using CT can be performed with as low mAs (20 mAs) as possible due to the contrast of bone and air, and hence the dose will be almost equal to plain films (Aalokken, 2003; Hagtvedt, 2003). Though MR can demonstrate the anatomy, CT is superior to delineate the bony details, as well as depicting soft tissue masses, in addition the surgeons always use CT as a surgical map.

The only patient preparation needed prior to CT and MR examination is nose blowing. Nasal spray with decongestants prior to examination is not needed. In order to delineate bony anatomy most properly, the patient should be in the prone position at CT in order let fluid drain away from the sinus openings, also referred to as the ostiomeatal complex (OMC) (Babbel, 1991). In acute recurrent rhinosinusitis imaging could favourable be postponed for some weeks for better delineation of the bony details when the soft tissue masses are less pronounced.

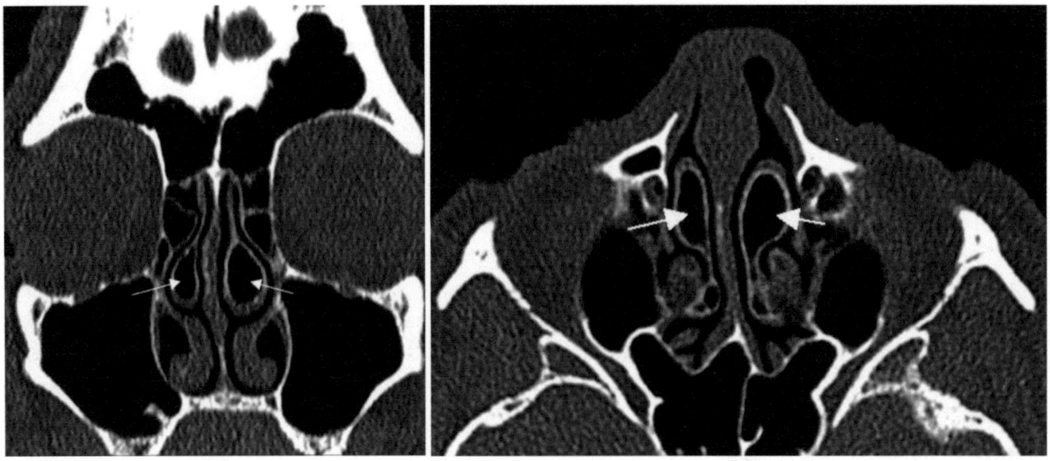

(a) (b)

Fig. 1. CT is the primary modality in sinonasal imaging. (a) Coronal CT through the anterior paranasal sinuses with the maxillary, anterior ethmoid including bilateral concha bullosa (arrows) and the frontal sinuses. (b) Axial CT through sphenoid, maxillary and ethmoid sinuses with bilateral concha bullosa (arrows).

3. Paranasal sinus development, anatomical and pneumatisation variants

It is mandatory for a correct imaging report that the radiologist is familiar with the development of the paranasal sinuses and recognises the bony variants and their influence on the mucociliary drainage routes.

The paranasal sinuses develop from fetal life till the nearly adult size by the age of 12 years.

The maxillary sinuses are present as evaginations from the nasal cavities at birth and show a biphasic growth with a rapid growth from birth till the age of six years. Then a second accelerated growth from the age of seven years takes place. Chronic rhinosinusitis in childhood may abort this acceleration of sinus development and cause maxillary sinus hypoplasia. On coronal imaging, maxillary sinus hypoplasia is easily recognised as the maxillary sinus floor above the nasal floor together with an oval shaped orbit and low ethmoid roof (Eggesbo, 2001b). The surgeon must be aware of this variant, because the uncinate process that is a bony landmark during surgery, is lateral displaced and the orbit can easily be exposed during surgery as well as a low ethmoid roof may expose the brain.

The sphenoid sinuses also develop from birth. At the age of six years the presphenoid is pneumatised and by the age of twelve years also the sphenoid bone below the sella turcica, termed the basisphenoid, is pneumatised. Finally, pneumatisation of the anterior clinoid and pterygoid processes may occur. The sphenoid sinuses have close relation to the cranial nerves, 3rd, 4th, 5^{th}_{I}, 5^{th}_{II} and 6th, and the carotid artery passing in the cavernous sinus and the optic nerve. When sphenoethmoid cells or pneumatisation of the anterior clinoid process are seen, the optic nerves are frequently inside the sinus and should not be mistaken for a soft tissue mass or polyp.

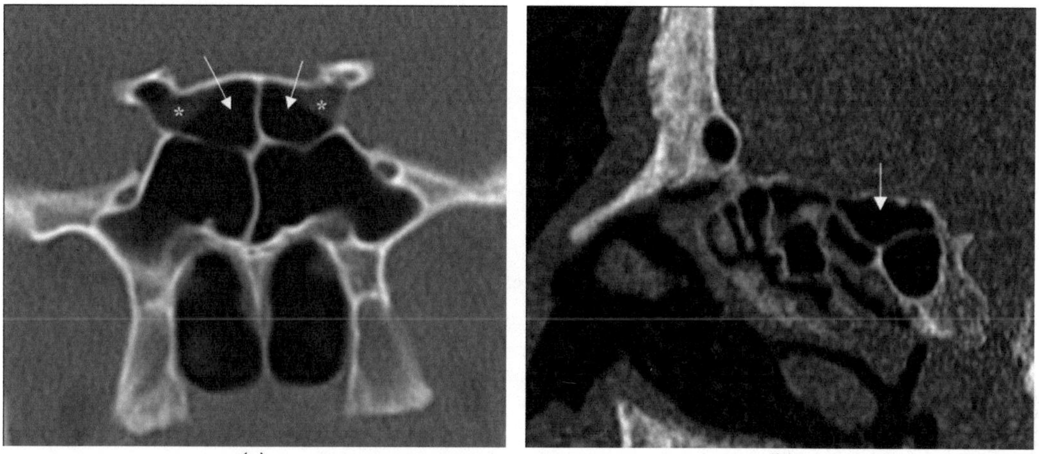

(a) (b)

Fig. 2. (a) Coronal CT through the sphenoid bone shows four cells, where the superior cells are posterior ethmoid (sphenoethmoid) cells (arrows) that have continued into the sphenoid bone superior to the true sphenoid sinuses. (b) Sagittal CT demonstrates a sphenoethmoid cell (arrow) superior to the true sphenoid cell. Also notice the optic nerves (asterisks) running through the sphenoethmoid (Onodi) cells in fig (a).

The ethmoid sinuses are developed by birth as fluid filled evaginations, and air-filled during the first year. Adult ethmoid sinuses consist of 3-18 sinuses (termed cells) on each side. The anterior and posterior ethmoid sinuses are divided by the posterior wall (Stammberger, 1995) of the largest and most constant ethmoid cell termed the ethmoid bulla (Latin word for bubble).

In a healthy person with no mucosal disease, the ethmoid cells may expand to the surrounding bone and form extra cells referred to as pneumatisation variants.

The most common pneumatisation variants from the anterior ethmoid cells are concha bullosa (pneumatisation of the middle turbinate), pneumatisation below the orbital floor and adjacent to the maxillary ostium, termed infraorbital cells or Haller cells (after the Swiss biologist Albrecht von Haller in 1743 (1708-1777) (Caversaccio, 2011), and agger nasi cells (pneumatisation of the most the anterior part of the maxillary bone). The importance of these pneumatisation variants is their close relation to the mucociliary drainage routes. E.g. a large infraorbital cell may obstruct the drainage from the maxillary sinus causing and infundibular inflammatory pattern, a large agger nasi cell may obstruct the drainage from the frontal sinus causing frontal sinusitis, and a large concha bullosa or large ethmoid bulla may obstruct the middle meatus and hence involve the ipsilateral frontal, anterior ethmoid and maxillary sinuses referred to as an OMC inflammatory pattern. A large ethmoid bulla may also obstruct the mucociliary clearance from the ipsilateral frontal, anterior ethmoid and maxillary sinuses.

The most common pneumatisation variants from the posterior ethmoid cells are posterior ethmoid cells that continue posteriorly into the sphenoid bone either laterally or superiorly to the sphenoid sinus, termed sphenoethmoid or Onodi cells. (after the Hungarian rhinolaryngologist Adolf Onodi in 1903 (1857-1919)).

The frontal sinuses are the last sinuses to develop and termed frontal sinuses first when the ethmoid recesses (sinuses) pass the superior orbital rims. This usually occurs by the age of six years. Aplasia and hypoplasia of the frontal sinuses is common, with aplasia seen in 5% of the population. A frontal sinus can be regarded as pneumatisation variant since its occurrence depends on the pneumatisation potential of the ethmoid sinuses.

By the simultaneous introduction of CT imaging and endoscopic surgery in the 1980's the pneumatisation variants were viewed as a main cause for rhinosinusitis. This is no longer the theory. Pneumatisation variants are a result of healthy sinuses that has greater pneumatisation potential than diseased sinuses. However, when pneumatisation variants are present, only a slight mucosal swelling can cause obstruction of the mucosal drainage route and cause rhinosinusitis. Therefore, removing the bony walls of pneumatisation variants, is an usual procedure when FESS is required.

4. Mucociliary clearance and normal mucosal variants

The paranasal sinuses are covered by a ciliated epithelium that beats with a frequency up to 1000 cycles a minute. The epithelium produce mucous that entraps particles and microorganisms and the ciliated cells clean up by turning the mucus blanket over every 10-30 minutes. The paranasal sinuses also contribute to humidify the inhaled air. Therefore, the mucous and fluid production of the paranasal sinuses can be as high as one to two liters every day. Each sinus has its own specific drainage route before passing through the ostium into the superior or medial meatus then passing to the choana. The anterior ethmoid, frontal and maxillary sinuses drain into the middle meatus and the posterior ethmoid and sphenoid sinuses drain into the superior meatus.

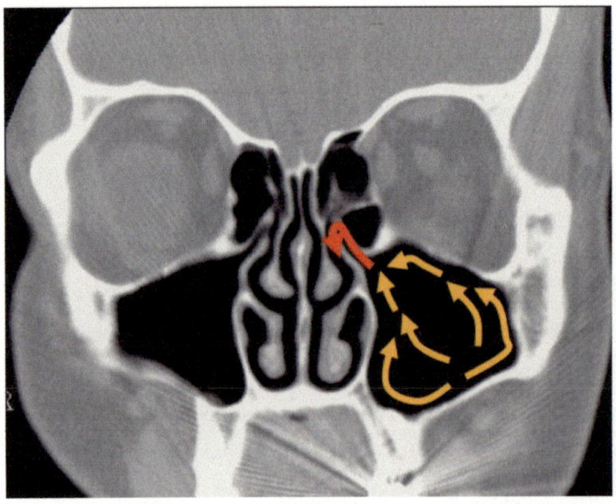

(a)

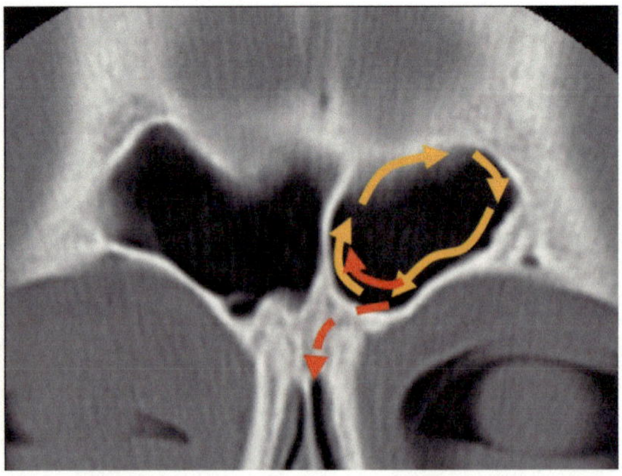

(b)

Fig. 3. Coronal CT demonstrating the mucociliary drainage route for (a) the maxillary sinus with it's final route through the ethmoid infundibulum (red arrow) and (b) the frontal sinus with it's final route through the frontal recess (red dotted arrow).

Swelling of the mucosal lining or polyps at the level of the sinus openings cause obstruction of the drainage routes and cause rhinosinusitis. One of the issues of imaging is to evaluate the patency of the mucociliary drainage routes and report on mucosal swellings and anatomical variants that may contribute to obstruction of these drainage routes.

In reporting paranasal sinus imaging the radiologist must be aware of normal physiological changes in order not to "over report" the normal findings as inflammatory changes. E.g. the nasal cycle first described by Kayser in 1889. The nasal cycle is a cyclical swelling of the ipsilateral turbinates and nasal mucosa. Unilateral enlarged turbinates are therefore a normal imaging finding (Zinreich, 1988). Also the ethmoid mucosal linings are influenced by the nasal cycle, hence mucosal thickening of 2 mm is commonly seen due to the nasal cycle and must not be reported as abnormal. Concerning the frontal and sphenoid sinuses the mucosal linings should not be visualised at CT, while maxillary sinus mucosal thickening up to 4 mm is often seen in healthy individuals and considered as a normal finding (Rak, 1991). With age, the nasal cycles become less prominent.

The nasal cycle, paranasal mucosa and mucous/serous production are regulated by the autonomic nerve system and neuropeptides from the primary sensory neurons. The complex system is still not completely understood, however it is known that the parasympathetic system and sympathetic ß-receptors stimulate secretion (Naclerio, 2010; Sarin, 2006).

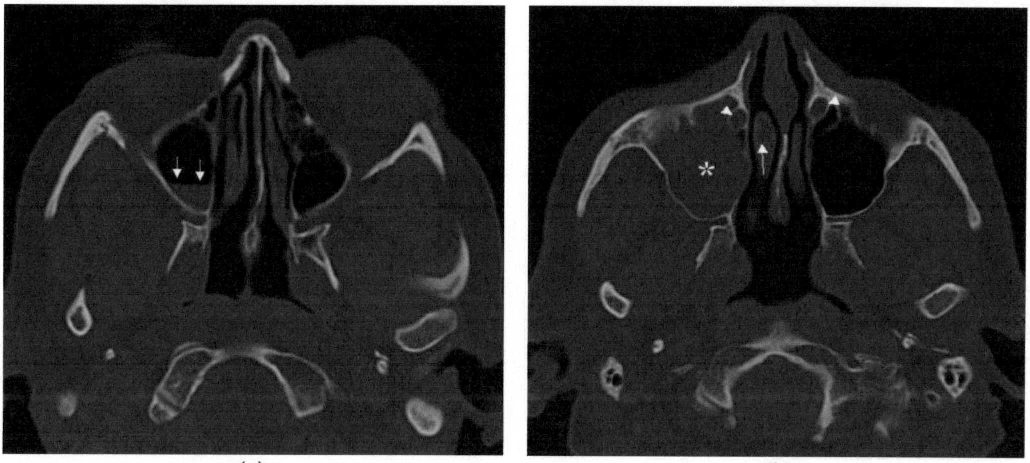

(a) (b)

Fig. 4. (a) Axial CT shows incidental finding of an air-fluid level (arrows) in the right maxillary sinus in a patient undergoing cerebral CT. There is no sclerotic bone thickening and hence no indication for follow-up. (b) Axial CT shows incidental total opacification of the right maxillary sinus (asterisk) without sclerotic bone thickening. Unless clinical symptoms of a acute sinusitis, no action to this finding is needed. Notice also opacified right concha bullosa (arrow) and normal fluid filled lacrimal ducts (arrowheads)

Primary sensory neurons releasing neurotransmittors can also cause increased mucosal swelling and fluid production. Finally, drugs that have a vasoactive effect can increase the thickness of mucosal lining and increase the serous fluid production (Cingi, 2011). Fluid filled sinuses can therefore be an incidental finding, especially in bedridden patients, and must be interpreted with care (Naclerio, 2010; Sarin, 2006). Air-fluid level is frequently seen in healthy patients and is not equivalent to rhinosinusitis. Only if the patient has symptoms of rhinosinusitis and the fluid contains air-bubbles, the findings can be interpreted as acute rhinosinusitis. The surrounding bone is a clue to diagnose chronic rhinosinusitis. If normal thickness of the surrounding bone a chronic infection can be ruled out.

5. Solitary polyps and retention cysts

Solitary polyps and retention cysts are common incidental findings in the paranasal sinuses and usually have no clinical implication. The maxillary sinus is the most common origin, especially from the floor of the sinus. Polyps are due to accumulation of fluid in the mucosa as are serous retention cysts, while mucous retention cysts are due to obstruction of a seromucinous gland. Polyps and retention cysts are seen as smooth, outwardly convex soft tissue masses at CT and MR imaging and cannot be differentiated. The MR signal depends on the water and protein content, and when the water content dominates, solitary polyps and retention cysts have homogeneous, high T2- and low T1-signal. If no underlying bony destruction is present at CT, the term retention cyst should be used and no follow-up imaging should be necessary.

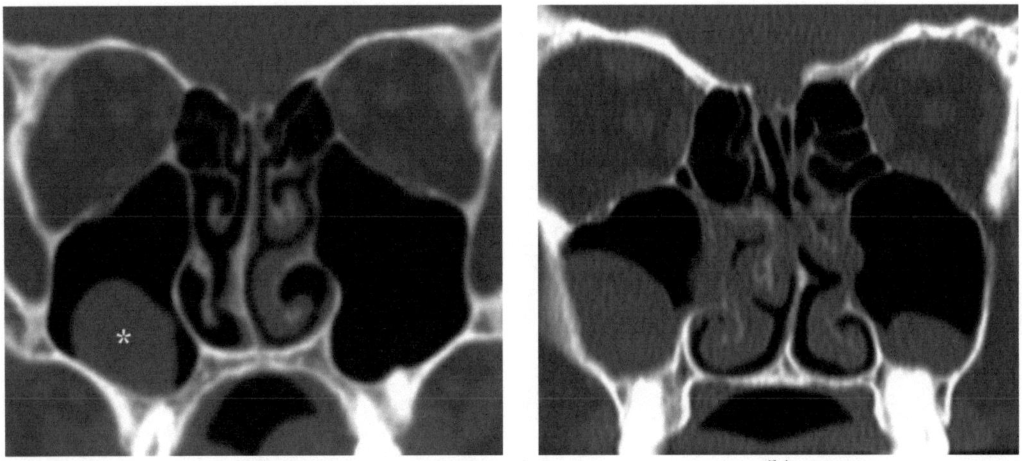

(a) (b)

Fig. 5. (a) Coronal CT shows a smooth, outwardly convex soft tissue mass (asterisk) originating from the maxillary floor. No underlying bone destruction or periondontic abscess are seen and the mass should be interpreted as a retention cyst. (b) Coronal CT in another patient shows retention cyst in each maxillary sinus and slight mucosal thickening/retention cyst in the right nasal cavity.

6. Inflammatory patterns

Five inflammatory patterns at CT have been described in chronic rhinosinusitis (Sonkens, 1991). These patterns are: 1. Infundibular, 2. Ostiomeatal complex (OMC), 3). Sphenoethmoid recess (SER), 4. Polyposis, and 5. Sporadic. The first three inflammatory patterns are caused by obstruction of mucociliary drainage routes.

1. The first pattern is caused by obstruction at the level of the ethmoid infundibulum, which is the drainage route of the maxillary sinus, and hence called infundibular inflammatory pattern. In this pattern only the ipsilateral maxillary sinus is involved.

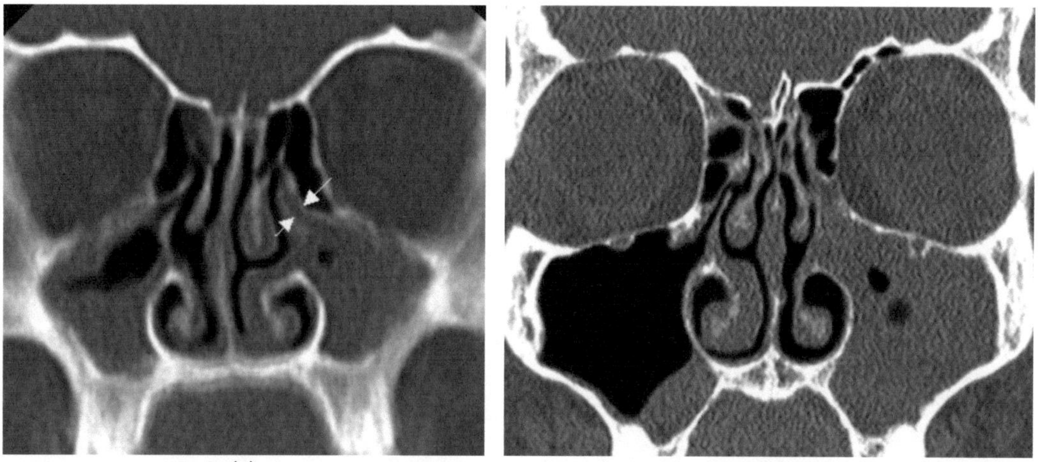

(a) (b)

Fig. 6. (a) Coronal CT shows infundibular inflammatory pattern with bilateral opacification of the maxillary sinuses due to obstruction of mucociliary drainage at the level of the ethmoid infundibulum (arrows). (b) Coronal CT shows unilateral left sided infundibular inflammatory pattern, and sporadic mucosal thickening in the right maxillary sinus floor.

2. The second pattern is caused by obstruction of the middle meatus, which is the final mucociliary drainage route of the ipsilateral maxillary, anterior ethmoid, and frontal sinuses. This pattern is referred to as the ostiomeatal (derived from ostium and meatus) complex (OMC) inflammatory pattern.

The frontal sinus drains either via the frontal recess directly to the middle meatus or through the anterio-superiorly aspect of the ethmoid infundibulum. Isolated frontal sinusitis is regarded as a variant of OMC inflammatory pattern.

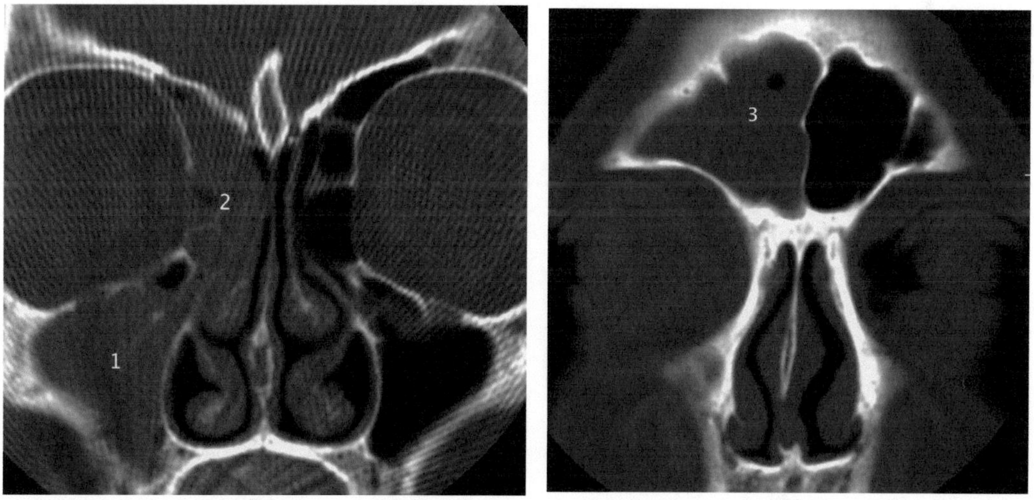

(a) (b)

Fig. 7. Coronal CT shows OMC inflammatory pattern with ipsilateral opacification of the (a) maxillary (1), anterior ethmoid (2) and (b) frontal sinuses (3).

3. The third pattern is caused by obstruction of the sphenoethmoid recess (SER), which is the drainage route of both the sphenoid and ipsilateral posterior ethmoid sinuses. An obstruction can proceed to rhinosinusitis only of the sphenoid sinus or also the ipsilateral posterior ethmoid sinus.

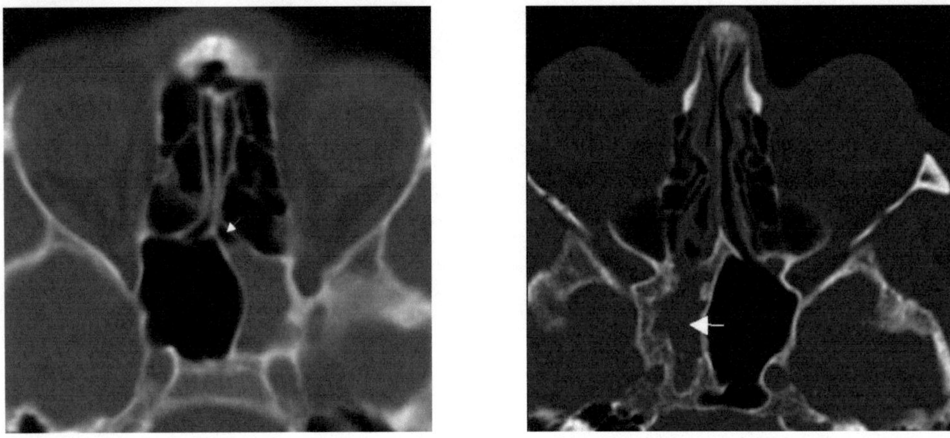

(a) (b)

Fig. 8. (a) Axial CT shows total opacification of the left sphenoid sinus with slightly thickening of the surrounding bone. Note that the left SER (arrow) contains air. This indicates that the obstruction can be at the level of the sphenoid ostium or the opacification can be due to a polyp originating from inside the sphenoid sinus. (b) Axial CT shows sclerotic bone surrounding the total opacified right sphenoid sinus (arrow), indicating a longstanding infection.

4. The fourth pattern is bilateral sinonasal polyposis and is characterised by enlargement of the ethmoid infundibulum as well as bulging and remodelling of the ethmoid sinus cells. In addition, the nasal cavities are filled with polyps, recognised by it's downward convexity contour.

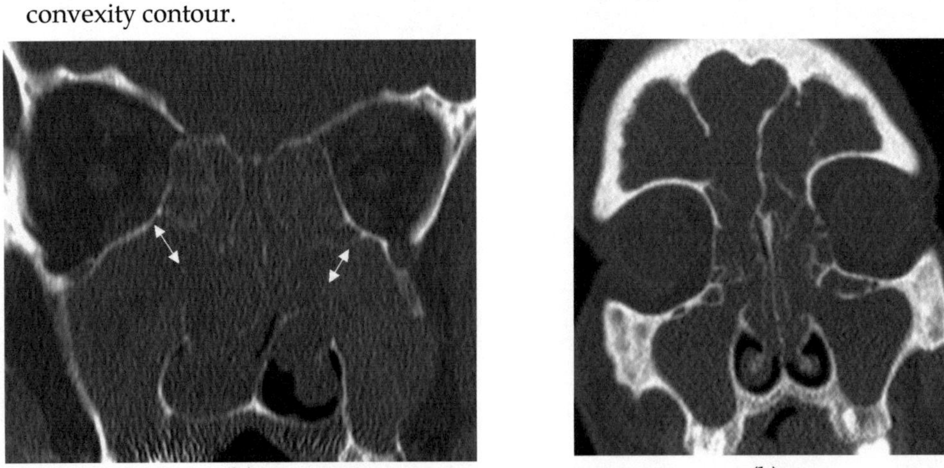

(a) (b)

Fig. 9. (a) Coronal CT of polyposis inflammatory pattern. Note the typical broadening of the ethmoid infundibulum bilateral (arrows). (b) Another patient where coronal CT also shows the involvement of the frontal sinuses.

5. The last and fifth pattern, includes all opacities that do not fit into the four previous patterns, e.g. solitary polyps, retentions cysts, mucosal thickening, and postoperative mucosal thickening etc. and therefore is referred to as the sporadic pattern.

It is important to recognise these inflammatory patterns in order to plan whether the patient will benefit from FESS, and if so the region and extent of the FESS procedure. E.g. In the infundibular pattern an uncinectomy or medial antrostomy alone will open the natural maxillary sinus ostium, while in the OMC pattern more extensive surgery including both medial antrostomy and anterior ethmoidectomy may be needed.

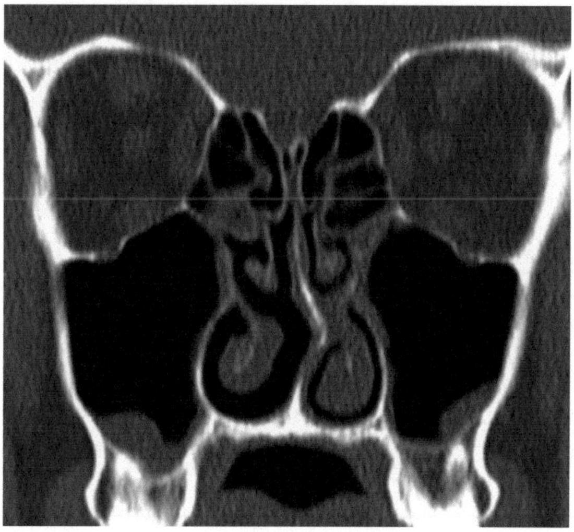

Fig. 10. (a) Coronal CT shows a retention cysts and sparse mucosal thickening classified as a sporadic inflammatory pattern.

7. Grading and monitoring chronic rhinosinusitis

In chronic rhinosinusitis, several systems for grading and monitoring have been proposed and evaluated. The Lund-Mackay system from 1997 (Lund, 1997) has been easy to use, however, all staging systems have shown limited clinical application (Zinreich, 2004).

8. Conditions mimicking rhinosinusitis

Many conditions may mimic the inflammatory patterns described and differential diagnoses must always be considered.

An antrochoanal polyp that occupies the maxillary sinus can be misinterpreted as an infundibular inflammatory pattern. The clue to the diagnosis is a small air-filled space superior in the sinus and soft tissue masses in the choana and with a polyp seen in the oropharynx.

Periodontal infection may cause inflammation to the ipsilateral maxillary sinus as well as the ipsilateral anterior ethmoid and frontal sinuses, and hence mimic an OMC inflammatory pattern. It is mandatory that the technicians include the maxillary alveolar ridge in the scanning, in order to rule out, or demonstrate an odontogenic origin. In case of dental filling artefacts, axial volume scanning will limit the dental artefacts to the axial plan.

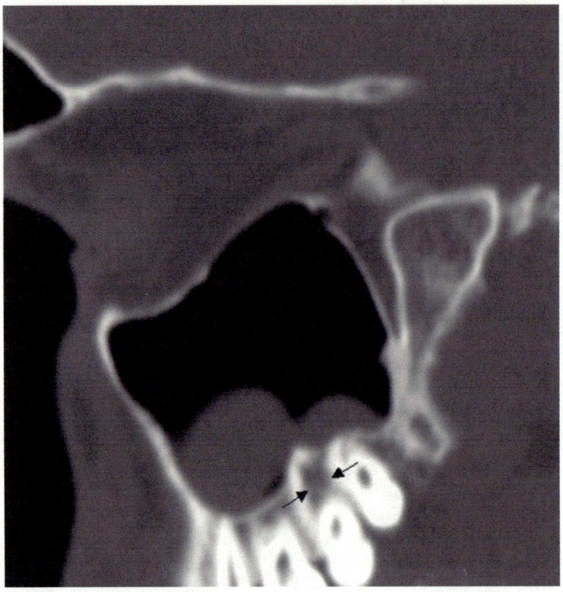

Fig. 11. Sagittal CT shows polypoid mucosal thickening in the maxillary sinus due to en underlying odontogen infection (arrows).

Rhinolithiasis is a rare and an under-diagnosed finding that is caused by mineralisation of an endogenous or exogenous foreign material (Yaşar, 2009). The patients usually present with a foul-smelling nasal discharge. When dental amalgam is the cause, the ethmoid infundibulum or the middle meatus may be obstructed and cause rhinosinusitis that mimic the infundibular or OMC patterns. Also an ectopic molar tooth free inside the maxillary sinus can give the same imaging appearance.

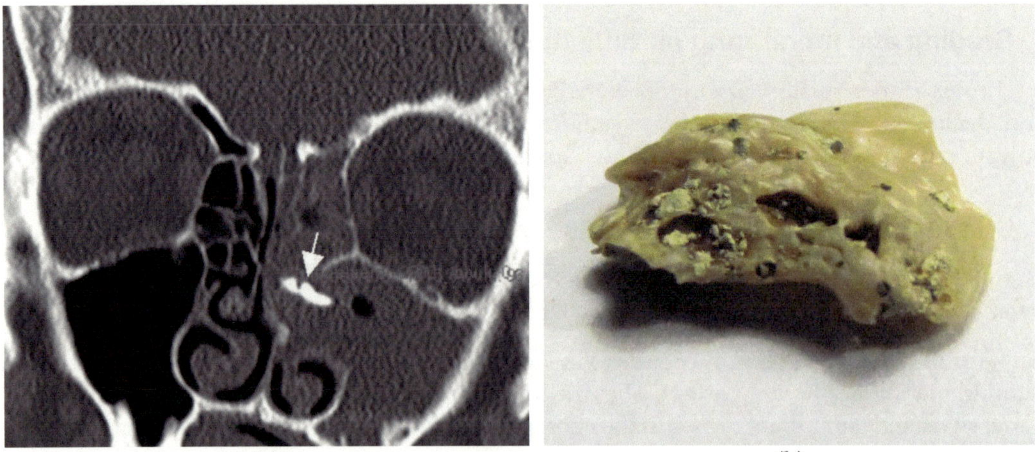

(a) (b)

Fig. 12. (a) Coronal CT shows advanced opacification of the left ethmoid and maxillary sinuses as in OMC inflammatory pattern. However, the inflammatory changes are due to an elongated calcification (arrow) located in the middle meatus. (b) A few months later, the patient delivered an ectopic molar tooth.

Several systemic diseases may show or present with sinonasal symptoms that may mimic or be equal to the patterns of inflammatory rhinosinusitis. The systemic diseases that may present with sinonasal manifestations are listed later in this chapter.

Fungal rhinosinusitis can imitate all five inflammatory patterns and must be considered in all patients with chronic rhinosinusitis. The characteristics of fungal rhinosinusitis are described later in this chapter.

Tumours are rare in the paranasal sinuses and contributing to only 1% of all malignant tumours. Therefore, malignant tumours are commonly interpreted as rhinosinusitis. All solitary nasal polyps should be considered for histopathologic examination. Destruction of adjacent bone at CT is one clue to suspect a malignant tumour.

9. Inflammatory complications

Sclerotic bone at CT is the most frequent response and complication to recurrent and chronic rhinosinusitis. Opacified sinus together with sclerotic surrounding bone should always alert the radiologist for the need of complementary MR imaging or follow-up CT. The thickness and morphology of the surrounding bone is an important clue to differentiate chronic from acute rhinosinusitis or parasympathetic dominance in a bedridden patient.

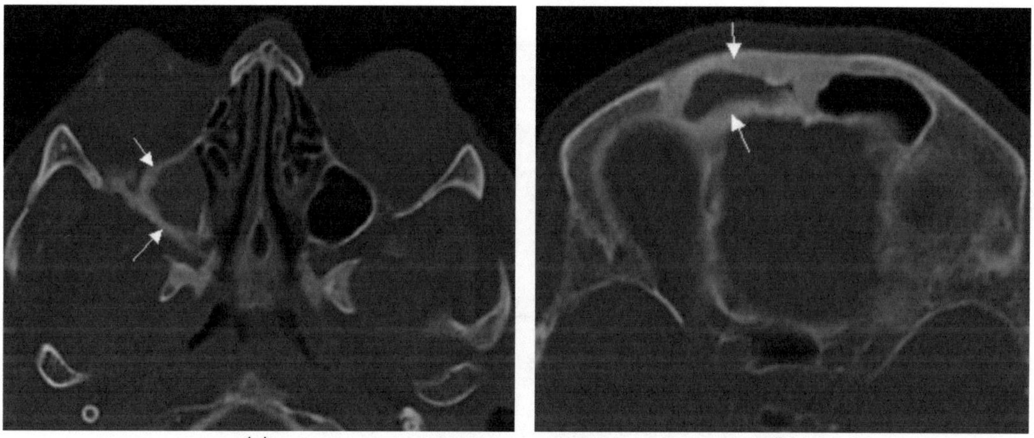

(a) (b)

Fig. 13. Axial CT showing total opacification of the maxillary (a) and the frontal (b) sinuses accompanied with sclerotic bone thickening (arrows) indicating a chronic infection.

Osteomyelitis is a rare complication to rhinosinusitis. Infection of the bone marrow of diploetic frontal bone due to frontal sinusitis may present with a subperiosteal abscess, commonly referred to as a Pott's puffy tumour.

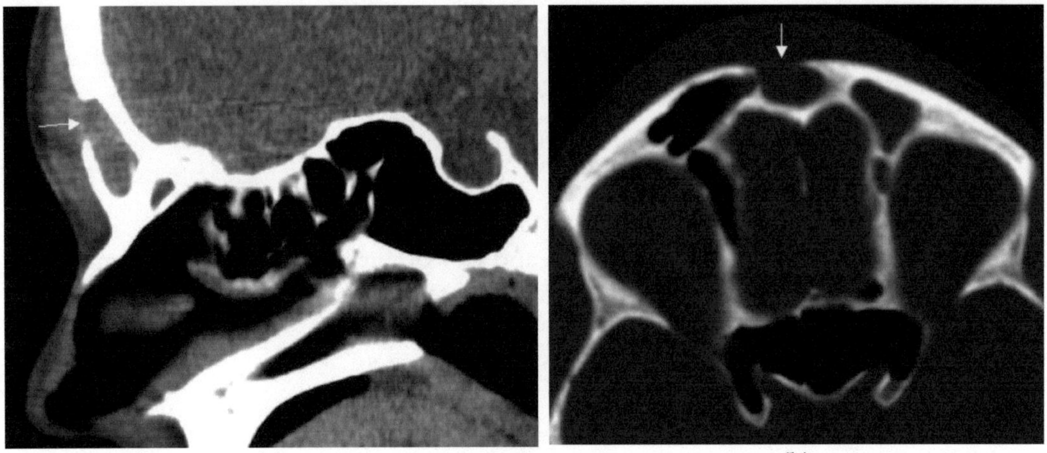

(a) (b)

Fig. 14. (a) Sagittal CT shows total opacification of the frontal sinus with erosion of the anterior wall (arrows) due to an eroding frontal sinus abscess, referred to as Pott's puffy tumour. (b) Axial CT in the same patient

Silent sinus syndrome, also more correctly referred to as chronic maxillary atelectasis, is a relatively newly described entity. The CT imaging features are almost pathognomonic with collapse of the sinus walls due to longstanding negative pressure, sclerotic thickening of the surrounding bone, and oval shaped orbit giving rise to the clinical finding of enophthalmos. (Soparkar, 1994). In this condition, the maxillary sinus volume is small, but should not be misinterpreted as maxillary sinus hypoplasia in where the molar eminence will not be pneumatised. Enophthalmos without the typical CT findings should not be misdiagnosed as silent sinusitis (Burroughs, 2003).

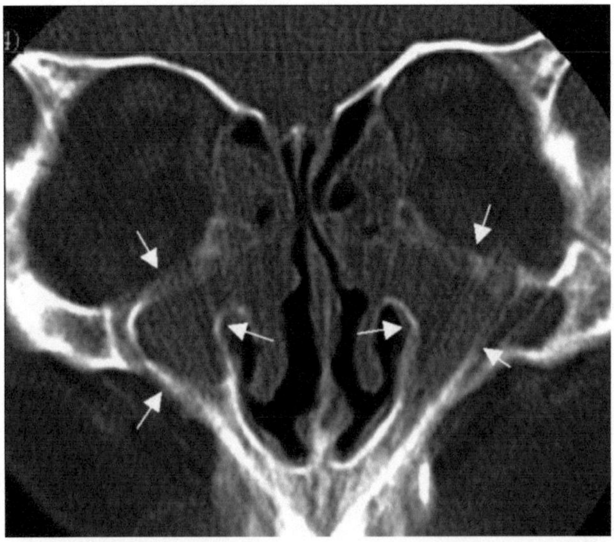

Fig. 15. Coronol CT in a patient with silent sinusitis syndrome due to bilateral, longstanding maxillary rhinosinusitis. The maxillary sinus volumes are reduced due to the inward retraction of the sinus walls (arrows). Note also the enlarged, oval shaped orbits.

Inflammatory spread to the orbits is more common than intracranial spread. I case of orbital abscess, the ethmoid sinuses usually is the origin of infection because the thin lamina papyracea and the ethmoid valveless veins easily allow spread of infection. Inflammatory processes in the sphenoid, maxillary and frontal sinuses, in descending order, are less likely to cause orbital infection.

Only 3% of cerebral abscesses are due to rhinosinusitis, with the frontal and sphenoid sinuses as the most common origin of infection, followed by the ethmoid and maxillary sinuses.

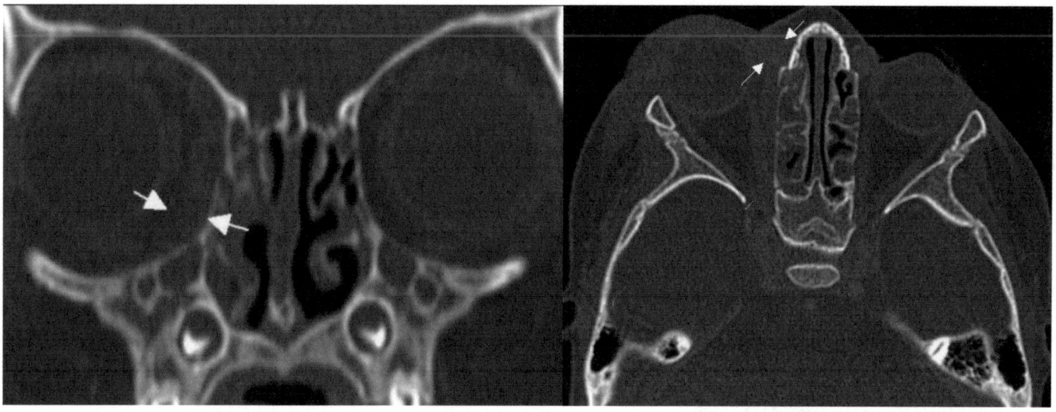

(a) (b)

Fig. 16. Coronal (a) and axial (b) CT show bilateral opacification of the ethmoid sinuses. On the right side there is exophthalmos due to spread of infection (arrows) from the right ethmoid sinus.

10. Mucocele vs. pyocele

Obstruction of a sinus ostium can proceed to formation of a mucocele, which is made up of mucous and desquamated epithelium. Over time, expanding of a mucocele will remodel the adjacent bone and sometimes also cause extension into neighbouring sinuses, orbit or cranium. Mucocele is most often seen in the frontal sinus, followed by the ethmoid and maxillary sinuses, while rare in the sphenoid sinus. When a mucocele is super-infected it is termed a pyocele.

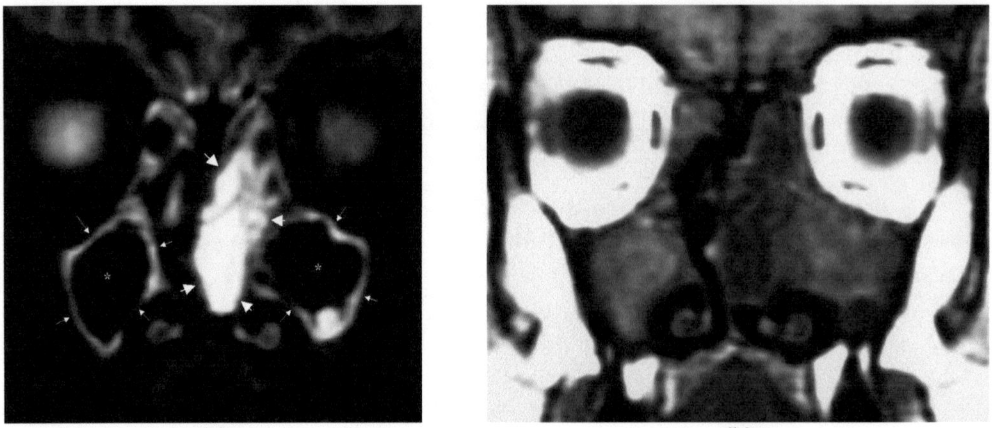

(a) (b)

Fig. 17. Pus-filled maxillary sinuses and a fluid-rich polyp in the left nasal cavity. (a) Coronal MR with STIR sequence shows bilateral hyperintense maxillary sinus lining (small arrows). and centrally signal void equal to pus (asterisks). In addition there is a hyperintense mass filling the left nasal cavity equal to a polyp (large arrows). (b) The complementary coronal MR with T1 sequence shows low signal in the mucosal lining and intermediate to high signal centrally, while the fluid-rich polyp has low signal.

At CT a mucocele and pyocele cannot be differentiated, though a pyocele tend to have higher density than the surrounding mucosa. Using MR however, the oedematous mucosal lining shows high T2 signal, surrounding a signal void or low signal centrally equally to the pus-filled lumen. The corresponding T1 signal is high or intermediate (Eggesbo, 2001a).

11. Atrophic rhinosinusitis

In atrophic rhinosinusitis the respiratory epithelium covering the nasal and paranasal surface is replaced by non-ciliated epithelium The primary form presents with a foul-smelling nasal discharge due to Klebsiella ozenae and widened nasal passages with a paradoxical feeling of nasal congestion. It is most common in young adults from developing countries as Southern Saudi Arabia, China, Africa, India, Mediterranean and Philippines

The secondary form is the most frequent and associated to previous nasal injury, surgery or inflammation (deShazo, 2011).

Atrophic rhinitis has become a more common form of chronic rhinosinusitis. However, due to lack of clinical criteria the condition is under-diagnosed (Ly, 2009). It has been suggested that the secondary form is a final common pathway following injury of the nasal mucosa Only a few papers describe the CT findings in atrophic rhinitis. These are nasal and paranasal mucosal thickening, small inferior and middle turbinates with atrophic mucosa and partial or total bony erosion. In addition small maxillary sinuses are described. This finding may be equal to "silent sinus syndrome" where chronic obstruction cause negative maxillary sinus pressure and with time the sinus walls collapse including the orbital floor, hence the patient may present with bilateral enophthalmos.

12. Sinonasal manifestations in patients with systemic disease

Sinonasal manifestations and chronic rhinosinusitis are described for many systemic diseases (Som, 2011), and may often also be the initial presentation of the systemic disease.

Cystic fibrosis

Cystic fibrosis is an autosomal recessive disease and almost only present in the Caucasian population. Though lung infections and malabsorption are the main clinical manifestations that usually are referred, all patients have sinonasal disease with mucosal thickening of all sinuses. In addition 40% present with additional polyposis. In CF children with mouth breathing and nocturnal snoring, a common finding is bilateral maxillary sinus pyocele. At CT imaging, they have characteristic medial bulging of the lateral nasal walls that totally can obstruct the nasal cavities. In these cases, a complementary MR examination will show peripheral mucosal thickening with high T2 signal and centrally signal void or very low signal equivalent to pus. The corresponding T1 signal is high or intermediate and will distinguish pus from an air-filled sinus lumen. The MR examination is mandatory in selecting patients that will benefit from surgery and to guide the surgeons to the pus-filled areas in the maxillary and ethmoid sinuses (Eggesbo, 2001a).

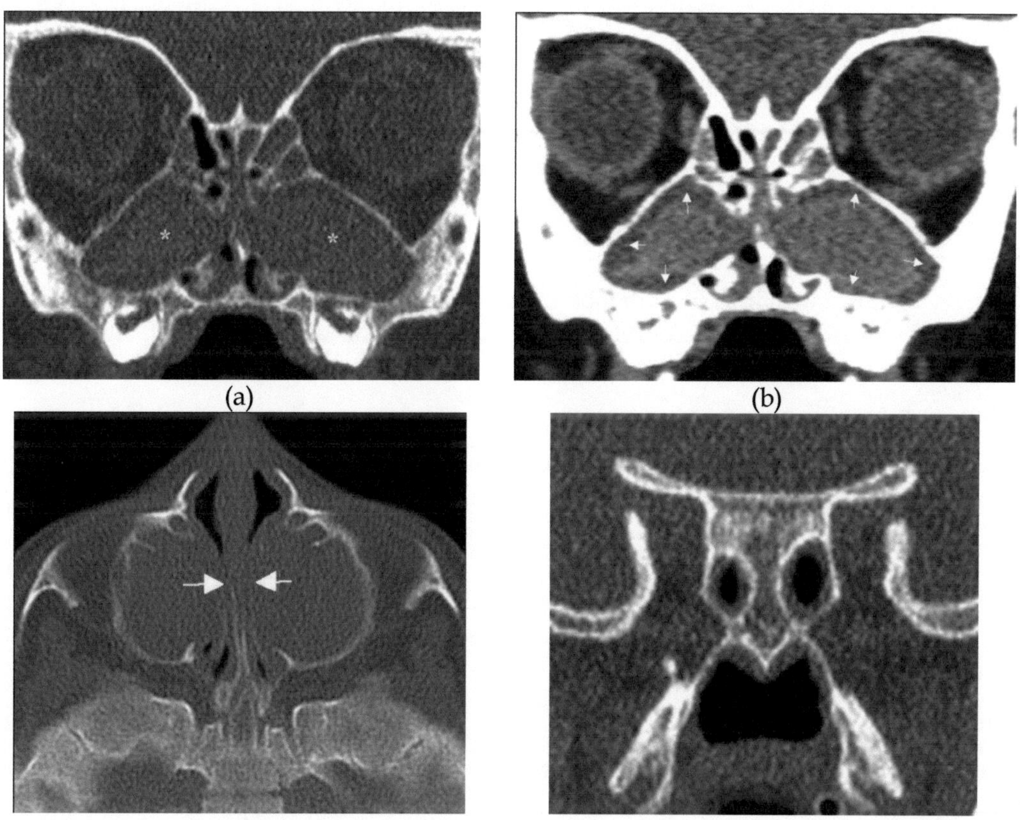

(a) (b)

(c) (d)

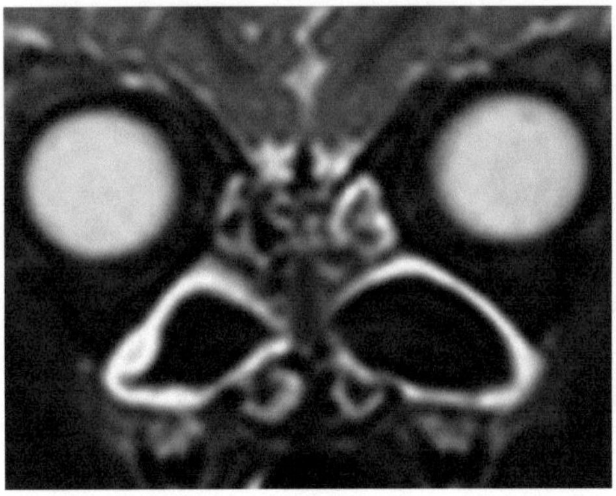

(e)

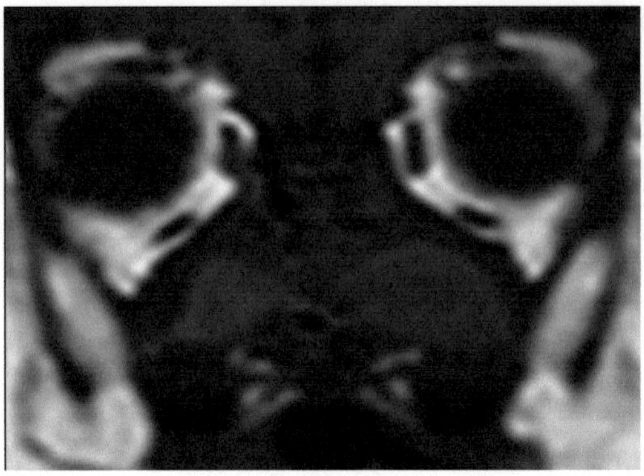

(f)

Fig. 18. Two-year-old boy with cystic fibrosis (CF). (a) Coronal CT with bone algorithm shows bilateral, homogeneous, ethmomaxillary soft tissue masses (asterisks). (b) Coronal CT with soft tissue algorithm can differentiate the mucosal lining (arrows) from the sticky mucous centrally. (c) Axial CT demonstrates the advanced medial bulging of the lateral nasal walls (arrows). (d) Coronal CT demonstrates sphenoid sinus hypoplasia seen in all CF patients. (e) Coronal MR with STIR sequence differentiates the mucosal lining from the pus-filled maxillary sinus lumen centrally. (f) The corresponding coronal MR T1 sequence is mandatory in order to discriminate the signal void lumen at STIR sequence from air-filled lumen.

Primary ciliary dyskinesia

Primary ciliary dyskinesia (immotile cilia syndrome) is an autosomal recessive disease with an incidence of 1/16000. The sinonasal manifestations are almost the same as in cystic fibrosis with opacification of all sinuses.

Young's syndrome

Young's syndrome manifest with obstructive azoospermie, pulmonary infections and chronic rhinosinusitis. This condition may also present with panopacification of the sinuses.

Sertoly-cell-only syndrome

Sertoly-cell-only syndrome with absence of spermatogones, bronchiectasis and chronic rhinosinusitis.

Hyperimmunoglobulinemia E syndrome

Hyperimmunoglobulinemia E syndrome is an autosomal recessive disease with dermatitis, skin infections, otitis media, pneumonia, impaired neutrophile chemotaxis, and high serum IgE and chronic rhinosinusitis is an usual finding.

Churg-Strauss syndrome

Churg-Strauss syndrome is a rare multisystemic disease, primarily in adults and with initial symptoms of asthma and allergic rhinosinusitis that cannot be differentiated from chronic rhinosinusitis.

Nijmegen's Breakage syndrome

Nijmegen's Breakage syndrome have microcephaly and variable rhinosinusitis and hypersensitivity to gamma radiation and hence, MR should be performed instead of CT, if imaging is required.

Aspirin triad syndrome

Aspirin triad syndrome in where the patients are hypersensitive to aspirin. The symptoms are asthma and chronic rhinosinusitis with polyposis.

Cyclic vomiting disorder

Autonomic nerve dysfunction is common in adult with cyclic vomiting disorder with sympathetic abnormalities dominating, while parasympathetic nerve function appears to be intact (Venkatesan, 2010).

Yellow nail syndrome

Yellow nail syndrome is characterised of thickened yellow nail, primary lymphoedema due to lymphatic hypoplasia, chronic cough, pleural effusions, bronchiectasis, and a propensity to develop malignancies. Chronic rhinosinusitis is seen in almost all patients.

PFAPA syndrome

"Periodic fever, aphtous stomatitis, pharyngitis and cervical adenitis" syndrome (PFAPA), probably on a genetic basis. This autoinflammatory entity also includes chronic rhinosinusitis.

Ataxia-Telangiectasia syndrome

Ataxia-Telangiectasia syndrome is an autosomal recessive disease or sporadic occurring with in immunsystem deficit leading to recurrent or chronic rhinosinusitis.

Weskit Aldrich syndrome

Weskit Aldrich syndrome is an X-linked recessive disorder where the patients from early life have eczema, bloody diarrhea and recurrent infections including rhinosinusitis.

Sarcoidosis

Sarcoidosis may present with nodules (non-caseating granulomas) in the septum and along the neurovascular bundles and chronic rhinosinusitis though rare, are reported as the initial findings in this systemic disease.

Wegener's granulomatosis

Wegener's granulomatosis (WG) is a necrotising granulomatous vasculitis involving the lungs and kidneys. However, the nasal cavity and sinuses are frequently involved and also may be the initial presentation with destruction of the nasal septum and lateral nasal walls accompanied by mucosal inflammation and sclerotic thickening of the paranasal bones. The findings at imaging may mimic postoperative findings and chronic rhinosinusitis.

Asthma and allergy

Patients with asthma and allergy commonly show polypoid mucosal thickening of all paranasal sinuses. Due to mucosal thickening also at the level of the mucociliary drainage routes, exacerbation of disease are commonly followed by extensive rhinosinusitis of both

OMC and SER inflammatory patterns. These patients also are more likely to have the sinonasal polyposis inflammatory pattern.

Gastrointestinal disease

In Crohn's disease and ulcerative colitis sinonasal mucosal thickening is a frequent finding, However, the literature is sparse about the sinonasal manifestations.

HIV seropositive patients

HIV seropositive patients rarely have rhinosinusitis as a part of the manifestations.

Cocaine nose

Cocaine nose presents with a hole in the nasal septum. In advanced cases both cartilaginous and bony septum can be eroded with destruction proceeding to the surrounding bones. The imaging findings are similar to Wegener's granulomatosis but the latter usually shows more irregular sclerotic paranasal sinus bones.

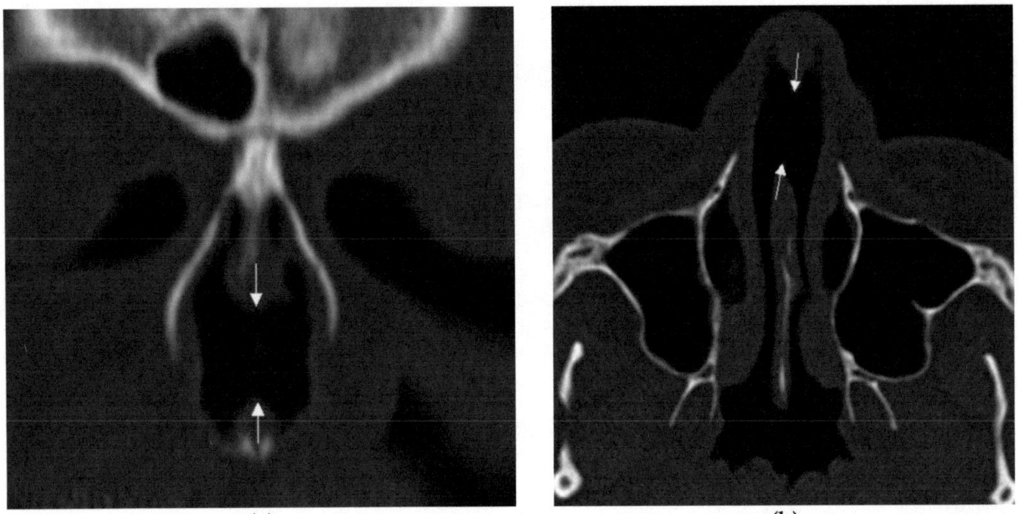

(a) (b)

Fig. 19. (a) Coronal and (b) axial CT shows a hole in the anterior nasal septum (arrows) in a patient abusing cocaine.

13. Fungal rhinosinusitis

Fungal sinusitis is classified as non-invasive and invasive. The two non-invasive forms are limited within the paranasal sinuses and consist of fungus ball (mycetoma) and allergic fungal sinusitis (AFS). In the invasive forms the fungal hyphae are found in the mucosal lining of the sinuses, in the bone and in the perisinus soft tissue. The three invasive forms are acute, chronic and granulomatous.

A fungus ball presents with foul-smelling nasal discharge. A typical CT finding is advanced unilateral sinus opacification with centrally scattered microcalcifications that are the clue to the correct diagnosis. At MR imaging the fungus ball has low T2 signal due to the microcalcifications, but also due to the paramagnetic properties of iron and manganese in the fungal hyphae. In response to the fungal hyphae the mucosal lining shows advanced thickening with high T2 signal surrounding the fungus ball.

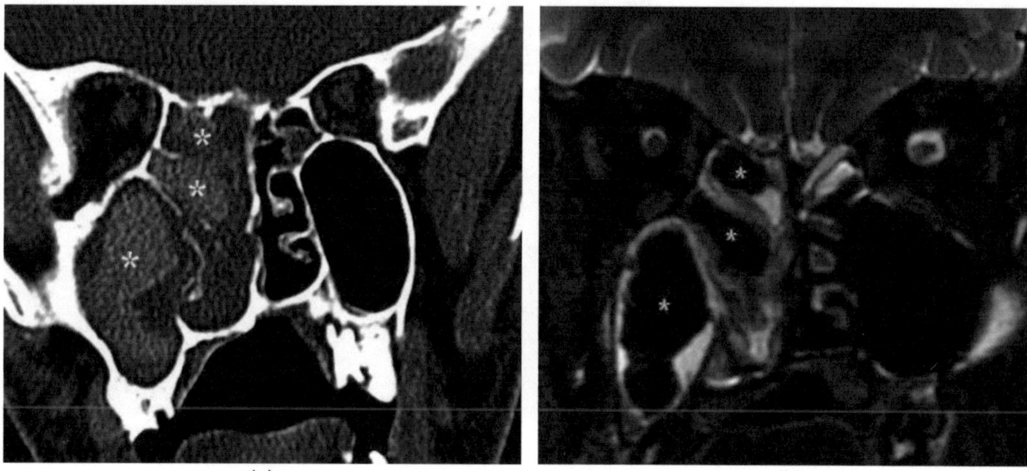

(a) (b)

Fig. 20. (a) Coronal CT shows total opacification of ipsilateral maxillary and ethmoid sinuses as well as the nasal cavity. The high density of the opacifications (asterisks) are a typical finding in allergic fungal sinusitis. (b) Coronal MR with STIR sequence shows signal void (asterisks) corresponding to the high density at CT. Courtesy A. ElBeltagi, Kuwait.

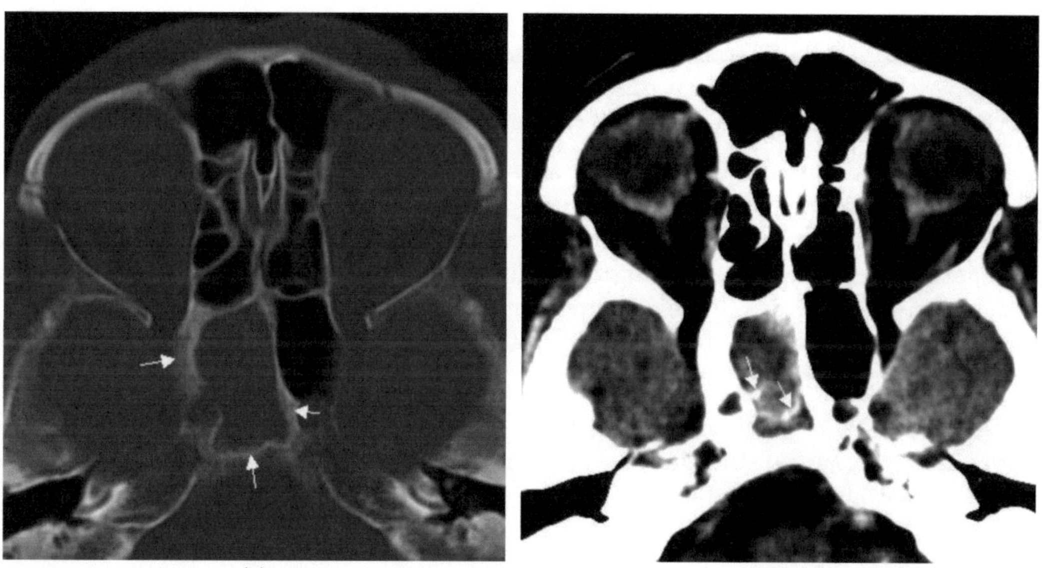

(a) (b)

Fig. 21. (a) Axial CT with bone algorithm shows total opacification of the right sphenoid sinus. The surrounding sclerotic bone thickening is equivalent to chronic rhinosinusitis (arrows). (b) Axial CT, with soft tissue algorithm reveals hyperdense calcifications (arrows) highly suspicious of a fungal infection. This was an incidental finding in a patient referred to cerebral CT, and missed initially.

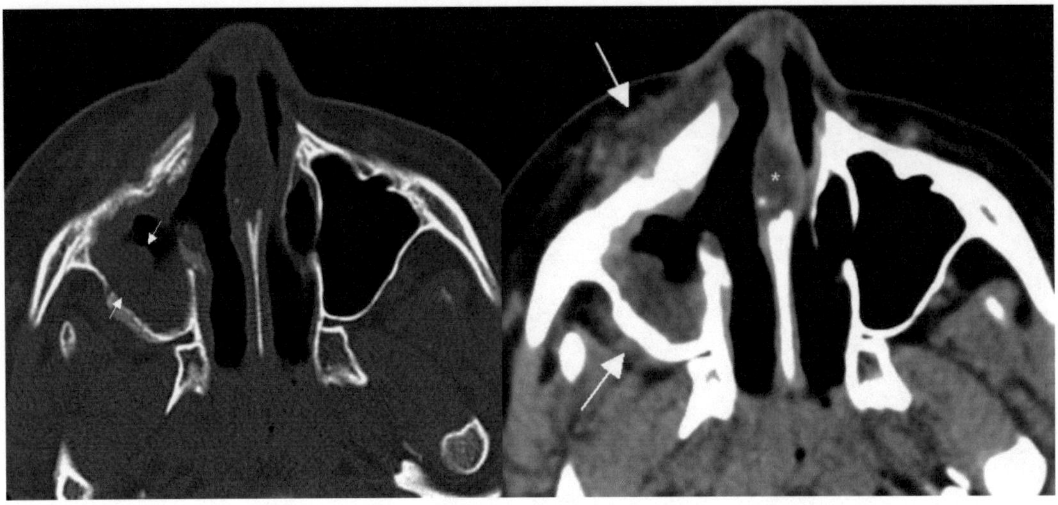

Fig. 22. (a) Axial CT with bone algorithm shows right maxillary sinus with advanced mucosal thickening (arrows) surrounded by sclerotic bone. (b) Axial CT with soft tissue algorithm reveals preantral and postantral soft tissue masses (arrows) due to invasive sinusitis. Notice also the septal thickening referred to as an eschar (asterisk).

Allergic fungal sinusitis is most common in warm and humid areas. The CT findings usually are extensive to all paranasal sinuses, but can also be limited to one sinus. The clue to the diagnosis is hyperdense central fillings surrounded by less dense mucosal thickening. The hyperdense central fillings is due to thick inpissated allergic mucin. At MR, the allergic mucin shows signal void at T2 and high or intermediate signal at T1.

In invasive fungal sinusitis, the acute and chronic form can be differentiated by its presentation. The chronic form can simulate chronic rhinosinusitis, while the acute form presents with rapidly progressive symptoms, while the granulomatous form is rarely seen. The clue to diagnosis of invasive fungal sinusitis is to look for obliteration of the fatty or soft tissue planes outside the sinuses. In invasive fungal sinusitis of the maxillary sinus one should look for preantral and retroantral soft tissue masses. In addition, a nasal septal ulcer may be seen, referred to as an eschar

In case of invasive fungal sinusitis from the sphenoid sinus the orbital apex and cranial nerves may be affected and the patient present with visual disturbances referred to as orbital apex syndrome.

14. Sinonasal tumour

Tumours in the sinonasal cavities can be extremely difficult to discriminate from rhinosinusitis in the early stage. In case of advanced unilateral opacification, bone destruction or bone remodelling, a malign neoplasm must be ruled out with complementary MR imaging. A malignant tumour may present as a single "inflammatory" polyp and therefore all polyps should be considered histopathologic evaluation.

15. The radiological report

Every patients referred to imaging may be a candidate for FESS, hence the report should start with developmental, pneumatisation and anatomical variants that may influence on the endoscopic procedure. The next step is to describe the localisation and extent of opacifications and to decide if it fits into one or more of the five inflammatory patterns described. Then most important when the patient has opacifications is to decide whether this is a "simple rhinosinusitis", then if there are complications to the rhinosinusitis, and last to rule out conditions mimicking inflammatory patterns, fungal infection, or tumour. In case of systemic disease, paranasal sinus affection can be sparse or mimic inflammatory disease, hence it is mandatory that the referring clinician includes sufficient information for the radiologist.

16. References

Aalokken, T.M. *et al.* (2003). Conventional sinus radiography compared with CT in the diagnosis of acute sinusitis. *Dentomaxillofac Radiol.* 32, 1, pp 60-2.

Babbel, R. *et al.* (1991). Optimization of techniques in screening CT of the sinuses. *AJNR Am J Neuroradiol.* 12, 5, pp 849-54.

Burroughs, J.R. *et al.* (2003). Misdiagnosis of silent sinus syndrome. *Ophthal Plast Reconstr Surg.* 19, 6, pp 449-54.

Caversaccio, M. *et al.* (2011). Historical review of Haller's cells. *Ann Anat.* 193, 3, pp 185-90.

Cingi, C. *et al.* (2011). Nasal obstruction as a drug side effect. *Ther Adv Respir Dis.* 5, 3, pp 175-82.

deShazo, R.D. &S.P. Stringer. (2011). Atrophic rhinosinusitis: progress toward explanation of an unsolved medical mystery. *Current opinion in allergy and clinical immunology.* 11, 1, pp 1-7.

Eggesbo, H.B. *et al.* (2001a). Complementary role of MR imaging of ethmomaxillary sinus disease depicted at CT in cystic fibrosis. *Acta Radiol.* 42, 2, pp 144-50.

Eggesbo, H.B. *et al.* (1999). CT and MR imaging of the paranasal sinuses in cystic fibrosis. Correlation with microbiological and histopathological results. *Acta Radiol.* 40, 2, pp 154-62.

Eggesbo, H.B. *et al.* (2001b). CT characterization of developmental variations of the paranasal sinuses in cystic fibrosis. *Acta Radiol.* 42, 5, pp 482-93.

Hagtvedt, T. *et al.* (2003). A new low-dose CT examination compared with standard-dose CT in the diagnosis of acute sinusitis. *Eur Radiol.* 13, 5, pp 976-80.

Lund, V.J. &D.W. Kennedy. (1997). Staging for rhinosinusitis. *Otolaryngol Head Neck Surg.* 117, 3 Pt 2, pp S35-40.

Ly, T.H. *et al.* (2009). Diagnostic criteria for atrophic rhinosinusitis. *The American journal of medicine.* 122, 8, pp 747-53.

M Som, P. &H. D Curtin. (2011). Head and Neck Imaging - 2 Volume Set: Expert Consult-Online and Print. pp 3080.

Naclerio, R.M. *et al.* (2010). Pathophysiology of nasal congestion. *Int J Gen Med.* 3, pp 47-57.

Rak, K.M. *et al.* (1991). Paranasal sinuses on MR images of the brain: significance of mucosal thickening. *AJR. American journal of roentgenology.* 156, 2, pp 381-4.

Rosenfeld, R.M. *et al.* (2007). Clinical practice guideline: adult sinusitis. *Otolaryngol Head Neck Surg*. 137, 3 Suppl, pp S1-31.

Sarin, S. *et al.* (2006). The role of the nervous system in rhinitis. *Journal of Allergy and Clinical Immunology*. 118, 5, pp 999-1014.

Sonkens, J.W. *et al.* (1991). The impact of screening sinus CT on the planning of functional endoscopic sinus surgery. *Otolaryngol Head Neck Surg*. 105, 6, pp 802-13.

Soparkar, C.N. *et al.* (1994). The silent sinus syndrome. A cause of spontaneous enophthalmos. *Ophthalmology*. 101, 4, pp 772-8.

Stammberger, H.R. &D.W. Kennedy. (1995). Paranasal sinuses:anatomic terminology and nomenclature. The Anatomic Terminology Group. *Ann Otol Rhinol Laryngol Suppl*. 167, pp 7-16.

Venkatesan, T. *et al.* (2010). Autonomic nerve function in adults with cyclic vomiting syndrome: a prospective study. *Neurogastroenterol Motil*. 22, 12, pp 1303-7, e339.

Yaşar, H. *et al.* (2009). Rhinolithiasis: a retrospective study and review of the literature. *Ear Nose Throat J*. 88, 7, pp E24.

Zinreich, S.J. (2004). Imaging for staging of rhinosinusitis. *Ann Otol Rhinol Laryngol Suppl*. 193, pp 19-23.

Zinreich, S.J. *et al.* (1988). MR imaging of normal nasal cycle: comparison with sinus pathology. *J Comput Assist Tomogr*. 12, 6, pp 1014-9.

6

Topical Membrane Therapy for Chronic Rhinosinusitis

Alan Shikani and Konstantinos Kourelis
Union Memorial Hospital, Department of Rhinology
Baltimore,
United States

1. Introduction

Chronic Rhinosinusitis (CRS) constitutes a longstanding disease process and a significant health hazard. Its pathophysiology may entail inherent epithelial irregularities, infectious insults, antigenic fermentations, and anatomic abnormalities, acting separately or in cooperation. Hence, various state-of-the-art treatment modalities have evolved, focusing on the surgical restoration of sinus homeostasis: endoscopic approach and visualization, fine surgical tools, power-instrumentation, precise imaging, combination of intranasal and external accesses, and navigation techniques. Despite the impressive technological advances in operative interventions, the medical aspects of CRS have not been investigated to the same extent, and the relevant remedies have changed very little over the years. Topical therapy in CRS is a relatively novel methodology, which relies on the local pharmacological management of sinus inflammatory status, and aims to supplement the existing treatment options. Topically applied medications have been used successfully for decades in dermatology, ophthalmology and urology. This chapter reviews the philosophy of topical therapy for CRS, its applications and effectiveness, as well as our institution's experience and findings regarding a complete local treatment protocol utilized for the management of refractory CRS.

2. Refractoriness of CRS and the rationale for topical therapy

CRS is one of the commonest chronic diseases, affecting 14.2% of the United States population (Lethbridge-Cejku et al., 2004). It places a substantial cost burden on the health care system and is responsible for a considerable portion of sick leaves and decreased productivity(Gliklich and Metson, 1998). The modern opinion points towards a multifactorial etiology which includes fungi, bacterial superantigens, allergy, aspirin sensitivity, exposure to environmental irritants, and lately, bacterial biofilms (Chiu et al., 2008). Moreover, conditions impairing the mucociliary function, such as primary ciliary dyskinesia and cystic fibrosis(Armengot et al., 1994) have also been implicated. The resulting chronic inflammation of the sinus mucosa leads to defense reactions and alterations, i.e. edema, high mucus secretion, cilia loss, and particularly, polyp formation (Meltzer et al., 2004).

Surgery to remove the diseased mucosa and open the sinus ostia in order to restore the physiological mucociliary clearance, in combination with systemic antibiotics, has been the mainstay of treatment for the past decades(Gosepath and Mann, 2005). The long-term success rate of endoscopic sinus surgery is reported as high as 76%. In the remaining patients, either no improvement is noted, or the CRS recurs soon after treatment. Interestingly, in the majority of failures, the post-operative sinus anatomy demonstrates ostium patency and wide-open ethmoid cavities, abundantly ventilated(Levine, 1990). Specifically, Kennedy has reported that 15% of patients who undergo endoscopic surgery, show mild to no clinical improvement, despite the "optimal" surgical outcome(Kennedy, 1992). These difficult-to-treat patients sometimes demonstrate inflammatory or idiosyncratic features, such as eosinophilia, history of asthma, allergic fungal sinusitis, nasal polyps, and aspirin sensitivity(Zadeh et al., 2002). The common denominator of the above conditions, is an intrinsic pro-inflammatory state of the sinus mucosa which predisposes to clinicopathological exacerbations, in the absence of substantial external irritation.

In addition to the aberrations of the end-organ, that is, the sinus epithelium, an unusual issue of resistance of ordinary bacteria to potent antimicrobials has emerged. This notable finding has been associated with the concept of biofilms, which cover the surface epithelium of paranasal cavities. The common bacterial species H. influenzae, S. pneumoniae, and S. aureus have been identified in biofilms, and their capacity to produce this organic matrix correlates with the refractoriness of CRS. Microorganisms colonizing the biofilms are much less vulnerable to systemic antibiotics which reach the standard tissue Minimally Inhibitory Concentration (MIC). Both the physical and chemical protection imposed by the organic layer on the microbial colonies, call for higher local concentrations of the antibacterial agents (Bendouah et al., 2006).

The principle of the local therapy is prolonged delivery of a highly concentrated drastic substance, whether pharmacological or not, to the sinus cavities, so as to exert its maximal effect on the desired anatomical site, without significant systemic toxicity. Oftentimes, the existing antibiotics and anti-inflammatory medications produce a temporary relief from CRS, combined with mild to moderate side effects, depending on the comorbidities of the patient.

3. Parameters affecting the efficacy of local treatment

3.1 Macro-anatomy

By definition, topical therapy should address thoroughly the target-organ, and reach all the subregions of the diseased paranasal cavities. Several patient- or drug-related factors influence the macro-delivery of medications, but the role of sinus surgery simply cannot be overstated enough.

The paranasal sinuses, have limited communication with the nasal cavity proper, and this is even more evident in the disease state, when the edema and mucociliary impairment further restrict the access to the inflamed regions. This situation changes dramatically after a successful endoscopic surgery. Even if, because of the aforementioned idiosyncratic factors, the CRS persists, creation of wide, readily-accessible surgical cavities is critical for the efficient local application of the therapeutic agents (Fig. 1). The frontal and sphenoid sinuses practically cannot be reached by intranasal administration, while a minimal diameter of 4mm is required for a slightly accessible maxillary ostium(Harvey and Schlosser, 2009). During an endoscopic procedure, the maxillary entrance can be opened as widely as 2.5cm, and the entire anterior wall of the sphenoid sinus may be removed. Regardless of the technique used for drug administration, the penetration in unoperated sinuses does not exceed 3% of the total volume placed intranasally(Hyo et al., 1989). On the other hand, radical surgical dissection allows contact of the drug with up to 96% of total sinus internal surface(Miller et al., 2004). Exactly how much improvement is provided by sinus surgery is difficult to assess though, as the various operative techniques are different in terms of intervention, and range broadly from minimally invasive (e.g. balloon sinuplasty) to extremely aggressive (e.g. modified endoscopic Lothrop procedure). Apart from the apparent gain in the total sinus surface contacted directly by the topical agents, clinical studies document as well that steroid sprays, when used by patients who had sinus surgery, produce more significant improvement of symptoms, endoscopical and histopathological findings, than in CRS sufferers having not being treated surgically(Lavigne et al., 2002).

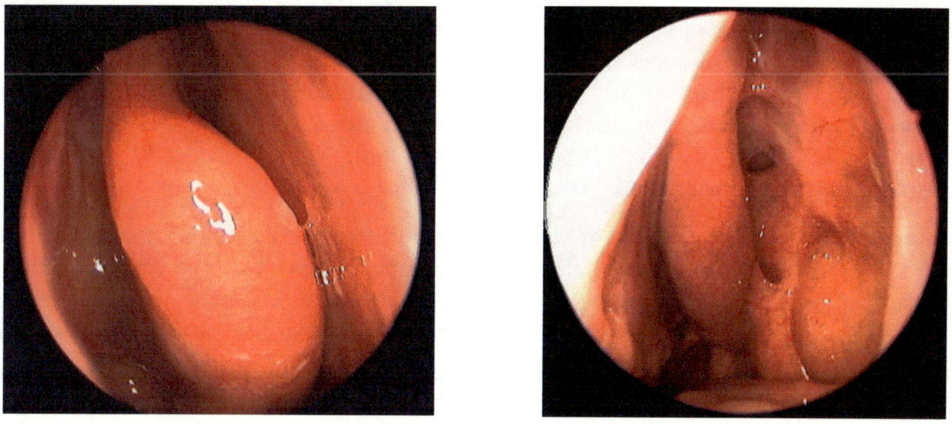

Fig. 1. In the unoperated patient (Left), the lateral nasal wall is an anatomical barrier to the delivery of topical medications, whereas the post-surgery paranasal cavities (Right) are accessible through wide windows.

Individual anatomical details, further modify the pharmacological penetration into the paranasal cavities. Inferior turbinate hypertrophy limits the intranasal flow, whereas in case of uncorrected nasal septal deviation, accumulation of the local agent immediately anterior to the spur is noted. Moreover, the variations taking place during the nasal cycle influence the temporal pattern of drug dissemination. Altogether, a patent nasal passageway, not narrowed by all of the above anatomical factors, permits 90% penetration rate of the locally applied agents(Unno et al., 1983).

A much debatable issue related to the delivery of local treatment is the patient's optimal positioning during irrigations or nebulizations. The traditional "Mecca" position with the head brought forward is becoming now less popular than placing the head backward. Lateral positions have also been proposed as more appropriate for delivery to the frontal sinus(Karagama et al., 2001).

A third consideration regarding the distribution of locally applied drugs is the configuration of sinuses in relation to gravity. Whereas the roof of the ethmoid and the frontal recess are dependent areas, so that the pharmacological deposits drain rapidly downwards, the maxillary antrum with its highly-situated ostium retains most of its contents, until they are cleared by the mucociliary mechanism.

3.2 Micro-anatomy

Even when the local agent enters the sinuses in sufficient quantities, its efficacy is not guaranteed, as it needs to reach its pharmacological target, and stay in contact for an adequate amount of time. This becomes particularly important in the sinonasal cavities, where the microenvironment is structured specifically to eliminate foreign particles, including medications, using several clearance mechanisms.

All sinus surfaces are covered by a mucus layer with the purpose to entrap foreign particles and filter the inhaled air. The production rate of the mucus fluctuates greatly, depending on the inflammatory status of the epithelium. Understandably, CRS is a condition predisposing to mucosal irritability and subsequent hypersecretion of thick mucus(Harvey and Schlosser, 2009). The thickness of the viscous gel phase of the mucus layer, which overlaps the respiratory cell cilia, varies from 7 μm in healthy mucosa, to 200 μm in high-grade inflammatory states(Tarran et al., 2001). Mechanical removal of the viscous mucus blanket, by high-volume sinus rinses results in more potent effect of locally administrated steroids(Daviskas and Anderson, 2006).

The mucus contents are as important as its physical dimensions and texture. Besides water, organic salts, enzymes, and immunoglobulins, the mucins constitute the basic ingredient of this supra-epithelial blanket. These are glycoproteins responsible for the viscous consistency of the mucus. In detail, mucins form fibers which bind to each other via cross-linking attachments, to make up a web that serves as the skeletal component of the three-dimensional layer. The mucin tangle contributes to the support of air particles, but also presents a network of hydrophobic sites, that act as receptors for macromolecules with similar physicochemical properties. Hydrophobic molecules are retained in the mucus and exert a prolonged pharmacologic effect(Ugwoke et al., 2005). On the basis of this finding, conjugation of topical medications with mucoadhesive gels, aiming to achieve sustained drug release, has been proposed(Nakamura et al., 1999).

In contrast with all the other Head and Neck sites, the sinonasal cavities are covered by respiratory-type epithelium, instead of the standard squamous-cell epithelial layer. Material that is captured in the mucus is gradually propelled outside the sinus cavities and carried to the nasopharynx, by means of constant ciliary beating. An intact mucociliary mechanism can clear the entire maxillary sinus of foreign particles in less than twenty minutes(Harvey and Schlosser, 2009). In CRS though, the chronic infection impairs the ciliary function, in favor of the prolonged residence of topically delivered medications. On the other hand, it is suggested that the active transfer of medications to the choanae might actually enhance their distribution to remote mucosal subsites(Goh and Goode, 2000).

3.3 Major delivery techniques

In the history of rhinosinusitis topical therapy, several methods for the delivery of the drastic agent have been utilized: Fluid irrigation, spray pumps, drops/powder/gel instillation, nebulization, and regional injection, aim to provide optimal spatiotemporal conditions of contact between the medication and its target.

Fluid irrigations remain a traditional, simple, and well-tested technique for conveying treatment formulas directly to the sinonasal surface epithelium. It is well-established that commercial nasal sprays, do not penetrate the frontal and sphenoid sinuses. On the contrary, a high volume of liquid solution (over 100mL) ensures access into these unapproachable sinuses. In post-operative cases, irrigations with a bulb syringe are superior to every other delivery methods, in terms of access to anatomical subsites. Yet, up to 30mL of solution pour out immediately from the nasal cavities, so that a considerable irrigation volume is wasted(Miller et al., 2004). Given a specific volume of solution, the pressure of irrigations can be modified by the device used. Low-pressure lavage using commercial pots, seem to be suitable for unoperated sinuses, whereas high-pressure douches delivered by squeeze-bottles are proper in case of surgically created open cavities(Harvey and Schlosser, 2009).

Nasal sprays have been classically used to provide local application of drugs in rhinosinusitis. Among the various devices developed over the years (spray bottles, aqueous pumps, dry powder atomizers), aqueous spray pumps are most accepted. Such pumps contain a medication-containing solution, which is released in the form of droplets. Smaller, lighter droplets demonstrate a broad distribution across the mucosal surface, as they travel a longer distance from the nostril. The viscosity of the solution is an additional factor, as thicker liquids project in a narrower cone and do not reach the peripheral intranasal regions(Kundoor and Dalby, 2010). Despite the refinements of spraying pumps, the droplets barely penetrate the sinuses in unoperated patients, and their effect is essentially restricted to the nasal cavities only. The maximal concentration of the sprayed agent is detected in the anterior nasal cavity, due to the obstructive mass of the inferior turbinate. Half of the dose does not approach the ostiomeatal complex, an anatomical structure central to the pathogenesis of CRS(Merkus et al., 2006).

Nebulized medications are a novel topical approach to rhinosinusitis, and have been used for the past decade in clinical practice in Europe. In Japan, they were adopted in 1950, and in the United States, nebulizers and nebulized medications are covered by most medical insurances(Vaughan and Carvalho, 2002). Nebulization devices provide an aerosolized mist which is created by a mechanical pulse. The latter is produced either by a high-pressure jet, or a vibrating mesh. The earliest devices emitted an aerosolized stream of particles larger than 10μm, and the penetration of medications into the sinuses was limited as most of the particles are filtered by macro- or micro-anatomical barriers. Innovative technologies are now capable of generating airflow consisting of particles with a diameter less than 3μm, and accumulation on sinus mucosa is much more extensive. The main advantage of nebulizers, in comparison with the traditional spray pumps, is the deposition of pharmacological agents in the posterior nasal cavity. Moreover, sprayed formulations are undetected in the sinus cavities of patients who have not had surgery, whereas 8% of intranasally placed aerosols remain in the sinuses(Moller et al., 2010).

4. Systemic absorption

The advantage of topical therapy is the accumulation of very high concentrations of medications directly at the target site. Equivalent doses would not be possible to be administered systemically, due to unacceptable toxicity. Nonetheless, the systemic absorption of locally applied drugs should be always kept in mind, so that potential side-effects are avoided. The nasal mucosa incorporates a rich capillary network, and certain substances applied onto the broad epithelial cover of the sinus cavities may reach high concentrations in plasma. The significance of drug absorption by the nasal mucosa is evident from the strong interest in the design of intranasally administered systemic treatments for miscellaneous diseases, e.g. diabetes (insulin), migraine (propranolol, sumatriptan), smoking cessation (nicotine), osteoporosis (calcitonin), and acromegaly (octreotide)(Ranade, 2001).

Orally administered medications undergo first-pass hepatic metabolism, and therefore a portion of the dose does not reach the systemic circulation. This is not the case in topical sinus medications, which are absorbed directly by the surface respiratory epithelium, and thus by-pass liver metabolism. However, the epithelial target cells of the nasal mucosa, contain an array of drastic enzymes, which also metabolize the pharmacological deposits. The levels of Cytochrome P-450, which participates in hepatic metabolism, are extremely high in the nasal mucosa, too. Phase II enzymes, like glutathione-transferase, which transfer micromolecular groups to the metabolized medications, are also prevalent. The nasal mucosa is deficient in proteases, though. Consequently, proteins are not lysed topically, and their absorption rate is substantial(Chien and Chang, 1987).

5. Agents used in topical therapy

5.1 Saline

Prior to the local application of therapeutic antimicrobial or anti-inflammatory agents, mechanical cleansing of the sinuses with saline irrigations has been one of the oldest and most widely used methods for the management of CRS. Mucopurulent secretions filling up the infected cavities are a frequent finding in CRS exacerbations. Furthermore, during the post-operative period following endoscopic sinus surgery for chronic rhinosinusitis, a collection of old blood, crusts, necrotic debris, or allergic fungal mucin, is accumulating periodically and regular meticulous cleansing is as important as the surgical procedure itself(Palmer and Kennedy, 2003). Office debridement, with the help of curved suctions is the optimal way to maintain sinus health. However, it is impractical and uncomfortable for the patients to visit the rhinologist too often for debridements as the only means of removing the "toxic" material. Our own policy is performing this debridement on a weekly basis, until the sinus cavities are clean. Frequent, as needed saline irrigations may be performed easily at home and are the simplest and least expensive form of topical therapy.

The appropriate saline concentration for the sinus lavage is controversial. Iso-, hypo-, and hyper-tonic salive, as well as Ringer's Lactate solution, have all been tested for their efficacy and side effects. Isotonic saline is the basic irrigation solution, as it provides only mechanical cleansing, without creating an osmotic gradient between the sinonasal cavities and the surface epithelial cells. It is suggested though that the isotonic concentration also modifies the rheological properties of the mucus, making the secretions less viscous. On the other hand, hypertonic solutions have been introduced subsequently into CRS management, as they decrease mucosal edema by creating an efflux of water from the intercellular space. Not only that, but it is documented that hypertonic irrigations improve the mucociliary function, in comparison to isotonic saline. High salt concentration in the sinus cavities is postulated to promote intracellular calcium release, which sets off the biochemical cascade resulting to cilia movement(Daviskas et al., 1996). Hypertonic sinus lavage also has an effect on allergic rhinitis, a major component of the CRS pathogenesis. Its main drawback however, is the discomfort often reported by the patients.

Apart from their chemical composition and salt concentration, a second characteristic of saline douches, unique in topical therapy, is the high volume of solution used in each irrigation. The importance of volume and pressure parameters has already been described.

Altogether, the benefit from saline irrigations to the management of CRS includes the mechanical removal of infectious/irritating/allergenic material, decrease of mucosal edema, improvement of the mucociliary function, and thinning of mucus secretions. Usually, saline rinses are prescribed in combination with other means of topical therapy, and there is evidence that they enhance the bio-supply of the primary medications(Papsin and McTavish, 2003).

5.2 Corticosteroids

Intranasal steroids have been initially the mainstay of topical therapy for allergic rhinitis. Due to their potent anti-inflammatory action, especially the deceleration of late-phase response, they diminish the manifestations of nasal allergy (congestion, rhinorrhea, pruritus). Their anti-decongestant properties in allergic rhinitis had been appreciated, and local steroids were subsequently introduced to the treatment of acute bacterial sinusitis, as adjuncts to systemic antibiotics. Interestingly, the infectious edema of acute sinusitis requires higher doses of steroids than those administered in allergic rhinitis(Moller et al., 2010). In CRS, local steroids were at first prescribed cautiously, and only in case of exacerbations, which resemble the pathophysiology of acute rhinosinusitis. It was the beneficial effect of steroids on nasal polyposis and hyperplastic sinusitis, that indicated their prolonged use in CRS. When steroids are administered orally, they have a clearly superior effect on nasal polyps ("medical polypectomy"), than any form of topical treatment(Palmer and Kennedy, 2003). Naturally, the advantage of steroid sprays is their capacity for long-term use with minimal side-effects. Perhaps the effective way to get the most out of corticosteroid therapy, is a combination of "induction" systemic administration to reduce the severe edema, along with a "maintenance" schedule of intranasal spaying, to control the continuous, low-grade inflammation of CRS(Wahl and Otsuji, 2003).

Local steroids are administered in several forms, in order to achieve greater efficacy. Intranasal placement of fluticasone drops has demonstrated a distinct benefit in patients with hyperplastic CRS, precluding the need for endoscopic surgery in half of the cases. The authors suggest that nasal drops are more successful than sprays, as they reach easier the middle meatus(Aukema et al., 2005). A modification of drops administration involves direct instillation in the office, utilizing a soft catheter, under endoscopic vision. This method accomplishes focused application in difficult-to-approach regions, such as the frontal recess(Palmer and Kennedy, 2003). A more invasive technique, combining the efficacy of systemic treatment with the low side-effect pharmacological profile of local drops, utilizes injection of steroids into the polyp mass. Although this procedure has been performed enthusiastically in the 1950s, reports of visual loss emphasized the need for cautiousness(Mabry, 1981). Embolization or spasm of the central retinal artery, have been hypothesized as the mechanism of blindness. Placing the injection into the center of the polyp lessens the risk of intra-arterial administration. Possibly, intra-polyp steroid injections do not have a role in the routine treatment of common CRS, but their efficacy could be useful in recalcitrant cases, not responding to oral or instilled corticosteroids(Antunes and Becker, 2010).

The chronic topical therapy with steroids has raised concerns of absorption into the circulation, and their well-known systemic effects: growth inhibition due to hypothalamic suppression, loss of bone density, hypertension, diabetes, and psychosis(Demoly, 2008). From each sprayed dose, 30% of the medication stays within the sinonasal cavities, and undergoes metabolism on the nasal mucosa, whereas the remaining 70% follows the oral route and is subject to hepatic metabolism. Altogether, the absorption into the circulation depends largely on the steroid compound, and ranges from 49%(flunisolide) to less than 0.1%(mometasone). A multitude of clinical studies has investigated the safety profile of intranasal steroids and no significant systemic side-effect was reported, either in adult or pediatric patients. Specifically for the latter, one-year duration of administration did not impede growth(Schenkel et al., 2000). Local adverse effects (dry rhinitis, epistaxis), sometimes causing considerable discomfort, have been documented, though(Giger et al., 2003). Interestingly, even in the case of intranasal injection, there is no clinical or biochemical evidence of adrenal suppression, although raised plasma concentration of the steroid has been noted(Mabry, 1981).

5.3 Antimicrobials

Unquestionably, microorganisms have a fundamental role in the pathogenesis of CRS, either by maintaining prolonged infectious processes, or by generating toxic allergic reactions. Antibiotics have been persistently used for acute and chronic rhinosinusitis, in oral or intravenous form. The rationale for topical administration derives from the concept of biofilm, which is clearly an "epi-mucosal" phenomenon(Lim et al., 2008). Among the various advantages that the microenvironment of biofilms provides to microorganisms is its poor penetration by systemically administrated antimicrobial agents(Stewart and Costerton, 2001). Moreover, the bacterial species found in biofilms, are no different from those commonly identified with conventional cultures in CRS (Al-Mutairi and Kilty, 2011). Interestingly, the minimal antibiotic concentration for the eradication of microorganisms residing in biofilms, can be as high as 1000 times their Minimal Inhibition Concentration (MIC) in the cultures from the same bacteria(Ceri et al., 1999). Therefore, chronic sinus infections refractory to culture-directed oral antibiotics was considered an indication for an alternative approach, which could overcome resistance by delivering high concentrations of medications in direct contact with the colonized epithelial coating.

The choice of antibiotic should be based on endoscopically-guided culturing of sinus secretions, keeping in mind the multi-pathogen etiology of CRS. When it comes to selection among drugs to which microbes demonstrate equal sensitivity, antibiotics that kill bacteria once they reach a critical concentration (concentration-dependent), like quinolones or aminoglycosides, may exert a more potent bactericidal effect, in comparison with time-dependent antibacterial medications. The latter, although effective in lower levels, require prolonged action at the target site. As already mentioned, the constant beating of the cilia propels the mucosal coating out of the cavities in less than twenty minutes. Thus, antibiotics such as penicillins, cephalosporins, or macrolides, which are first-choice systemic treatment options for sinusitis, cannot be considered ideal for topical therapy, due to their rapid clearance(Palmer and Kennedy, 2003). An additional factor influencing the selection of topical agents is their differential metabolic processing locally and systemically. Drugs which are deactivated promptly in plasma, but remain intact in the sinus secretions, are both effective and safe. Mupirocin belongs to this class, and is currently the only FDA-approved medication for intranasal use(Uren et al., 2008). With regard to non-bacterial causes of CRS, fungi are considered a prominent etiologic factor, in up to 90% of cases in several studies(Ponikau et al., 1999). Therefore, antimycotic agents, like amphotericin B and itraconazole, are promising local agents, since their chronic systemic administration produces serious adverse effects.

A few delivery methods have been tried for local antimicrobial therapy. Spraying of solutions with the use of atomizers, which is an efficient technique in the case of nasal steroids, has produced the poorest results. Small mucosal surface of initial application, along with the slow mucocliliary clearance which commonly accompanies CRS, possibly result in a limited area of drug deposition(Sykes et al., 1986). In contrast, sinus lavage with antibacterial solutions is more popular, and seems to be more effective as well. Frequent bottle irrigations with 300ml of ceftazidime, an antibiotic not available in oral form, are successful in eradicating Pseudomonas from patients with recalcitrant sinusitis(Leonard and Bolger, 1999). However, their efficacy may not be dependent solely on the proper delivery of the antibiotic, but also on the effects of the lavage itself, that is, the mechanical cleansing, dilution of mucus, and decrease of mucosal edema(Lim et al., 2008). A more advanced irrigation technique, employing endoscopic catheterization of the middle meatus, has achieved the resolution of CRS in the morbid context of cystic fibrosis. Yet, this modification of sinus rinsing requires frequent office visits, and interferes with patient compliance(Moss and King, 1995). Nebulization of antibiotics has emerged as both an effective and convenient delivery method. When the size of aerosolized particles is optimized to less than 5μm, this form of topical antimicrobial therapy is superior even to IV mode of administration. Similar to the case of antibiotic irrigations, an additional, non anti-infectious, beneficial mechanism of the aerosolized stream was postulated. Possibly, nebulization into the sinonasal cavities promotes anti-inflammatory and anti-edematous effects(Lim et al., 2008).

The findings from studies investigating the efficacy of topical antimicrobial therapy, are quite encouraging. Up to 88% of patients experience significant improvement, good quality of life, and few local side effects (rhinitis), after four weeks of treatment(Vaughan and Carvalho, 2002). This symptomatic relief is concurrent with reversal of the endoscopic findings. Refractory infections by resistant strains of Staphylococcus aureus in particular, respond dramatically to irrigations with mupirocin solution(Uren et al., 2008). On the other hand, topical application of antifungal agents did not produce a distinct therapeutic result in the management of CRS(Weschta et al., 2004). This finding is not in agreement with the hypothesis that fungal infection accounts for the majority of chronic sinusitis. Since fungi are ubiquitous in the environment and the sinus cavities, they seem impossible to be eradicated simply by local administration of antimycotic drugs. In the case of CRS induced by fungi, the pathogenesis entails an immune host reaction against fungal antigens, and as a result, inflammatory modifiers might be more appropriate than any anti-infectious remedy(Lim et al., 2008).

5.4 Mucoactive agents

As stated previously, biofilms may alter significantly the pathophysiology of CRS and protect the pathogens from systemic or local treatments, thus perpetuating the infection. Not only that, but it is suggested that this bioorganic coating acts as a reservoir of bacteria, and releases microorganisms in the conventional "planktonik" form, into the sinus cavity(Al-Mutairi and Kilty, 2011). Obviously, novel approaches to refractory sinusitis cases, focus on the elimination of this enigmatic entity. Being a distinct structure, analogous to a foreign body, biofilm is an ideal target for topical therapy, as the regional vasculature might not deliver sufficient amounts of systemic medications to the interface between the epithelium and the colonized structure.

Surfactants are ampthipathic compounds, that is, they possess both hydrophilic and lipophilic properties. Consequently, they are soluble both to water and organic substances. The well-known pulmonary surfactant decreases the adhesiveness of sputum to the lung respiratory epithelium, and facilitates the removal of mucus from the lung parenchyma. It is hypothesized that in a similar fashion, intranasally administered surfactants interfere with the adherence of the biofilm layer to the underlying sinus epithelium(Suh et al., 2010). This would result in biofilm peeling off the sinus walls, and the transition of recalcitrant CRS to a less complicated form, amenable to treatment. This scenario has been clinically tested in patients irrigating with baby shampoo, an inexpensive, nontoxic mixture of various surfactants. Almost half of the patients reported a marked improvement in their "mucus-related" symptoms, i.e. thick nasal discharge and post-nasal drip(Chiu et al., 2008). Secondary effects of surfactants have also been postulated, such as destabilization of bacterial membranes with leaking of electrolytes.

A promising local agent, due to its safety profile and low cost, is honey. In vitro testing documented eradication of Staphylococcus aureus and Pseudomonas aeruginosa in biofilm colonies, after treatment with several types of honey. Notably, honey was effective even against Methicillin Resistant Staphylococcus Aureus (MRSA), which is considered a plague of our time(Alandejani et al., 2009). The exact antimicrobial and mucoactive properties of honey are yet to be discovered.

5.5 Decongestants

Intranasal decongestants are the most frequently local agents used by sinusitis patients (16%) in the United States, more often even than local steroids. Perhaps the high prevalence of use can be explained by their availability over the counter, as well as the rapid, almost immediate, relief they provide from nasal congestion. Physicians usually prescribe a short-term course of decongestant sprays only in cases of severe, acute exacerbations of CRS(Sharp et al., 2007). Local decongestants are sympathomimetic agonists, which stimulate alpha-adrenergic receptors on the smooth-muscle fibers of the vessels beneath the nasal respiratory epithelium. As a result, brisk, potent vasoconstriction ensues. Interestingly, local sympathomimetics and steroids produce decongestion via different mechanisms, so that an additive effect could be accomplished by concurrent use of the two medications(Yoo et al., 1997). Although vasoactive decongestants reverse fast and effectively the mucosal edema, their local complications (rebound congestion, dry rhinitis, epistaxis) preclude their chronic use(Eccles et al., 2008).

5.6 Antihistamines

Antihistamines do not treat rhinosinusitis per se, but they alleviate the mucosal inflammation of allergic rhinitis. Although allergic rhinitis reasonably seems a predisposing factor for CRS, a direct etiologic relationship has not been demonstrated. Nonetheless, the incidence of CRS is higher in patients with allergic rhinitis or atopy. Furthermore, chronic sinusitis in the setting of allergic rhinitis is more resistant either to medical or surgical treatment, than the CRS variant of the non-allergic population(Krouse, 2000). Therefore, antihistamines could be incorporated into the management plan of selected CRS cases. Systemic antihistamines have been traditionally used in allergic rhinitis, with certain central nervous side-effects, such as sedation, poor attention, and impaired school or work performance.

Aiming to achieve maximum therapeutic action, as well as a lower rate of adverse effects, intranasally sprayed antihistamines are now included in the treatment armamentarium. Topical agents (azelastine, olopatadine) have shown indeed superior efficacy and safer profile than oral antihistamines. Moreover, they have the fastest onset of action (15 minutes for azelastine), among all the drugs administered for rhinitis, whether systemically or topically(Horak and Zieglmayer, 2009). Olopatadine, is well tolerated in children without causing somnolence, or compromising school performance(Berger et al., 2009). Interestingly, azelastine, besides blocking H1-receptors, exerts a few anti-inflammatory effects, e.g. mast-cell stabilization, inhibition of Tumor Necrosis Factor-alpha, and reduction of pro-inflammatory cytokines. Thus, it is effective in both allergic and non-allergic rhinitis(Horak and Zieglmayer, 2009).

6. Our experience in topical CRS therapy

6.1 The rhinotopic protocol: Why we do it

As already mentioned, chronic rhinosinusitis is persistent and symptomatic even after optimal medical or surgical management, in 5-25% of cases. In spite of widely open sinus cavities that are ventilated and drain readily to the nasal cavity, the mucosa is still inflamed and edematous, often with gross polyposis. We suspect that this variant of CRS is a medical disease, and the element of surgical obstruction is not the key pathogenetic factor. The sinus mucosa itself may be inherently predisposed to sustained inflammation, and in that case, it should be the target of pharmacological interventions. Even when these patients receive maximal standard medical treatment, sinus inflammation responds poorly or temporarily, and relapses are very common.

Consequently, patients undergo multiple surgical procedures, essentially for polyp debulking only, receive high doses of systemic steroids or potent antibiotics, and follow long courses of immunotherapy or desensitization therapy to address the allergic component of rhinosinusitis. Chronic or recurrent severe symptoms, impose a considerable cost burden due to multiple ineffective treatment attempts, but also impair dreadfully the quality of life. The frustration that patients naturally experience, introduces the "psycho-sinus" component to the natural history of refractory CRS. Typically, patients are fatigued, depressed and express their hopelessness. They confront the rhinologist with their feelings of disappointment and questions about new promising therapies, whereas they soon become non-compliant with the physician's instructions. The emotional distress of CRS sufferers is more debilitating than that of more severe, life-threatening chronic illnesses, such as congestive heart failure and chronic obstructive pulmonary disease(Gliklich and Metson, 1995).

The rhinotopic protocol is a comprehensive form of topical therapy for CRS unresponsive to standard regimens. It focuses on sinus membrane therapy, and aims to provide long-term alleviation of symptoms, with minimal discomfort and adverse effects.

6.2 The rhinotopic protocol: How we do it

The rhinotopic protocol originated in our rhinology practice, in a teaching community hospital. Moreover, patients follow a thorough treatment regimen at home(Shikani et al., 2010).

6.2.1 Patients

Inclusion criteria:

1. Previous endoscopic sinus surgery.
2. Recurrent or chronic sinusitis symptoms.
3. Endoscopic and radiologic evidence of sinus mucosal thickening or polyps.
4. Endoscopic and radiologic evidence of patent sinus ostia.
5. Trial of at least 2 courses of oral antimicrobial treatment without significant improvement.
6. Prolonged use of standard local treatments (saline irrigations, intranasal steroid sprays, intranasal decongestants)

Exclusion criteria:

1. Minor (<18 years of age).
2. Patient above 80 years of age.
3. Pregnant and breastfeeding women.
4. Allergy to specific antibiotics.
5. Patient currently taking oral corticosteroids.
6. Patient currently taking oral antibiotics.

6.2.2 Protocol design

The rhinotopic protocol is a strictly local form of CRS therapy, and does not involve administration of any systemic medications at any point. Two weeks prior to the beginning of treatment, a swab aerobic & anaerobic culture is taken endoscopically from the middle meatus to determine the dominant microorganism(s). Under local anesthesia, a piece of diseased mucosa is excised for histopathological assessment, as well as identification and quantification of the supra-epithelial biofilm layer.

The patients follow a 6-week regimen at home, consisting of saline irrigations twice a day, followed by intranasal aerosolization (Fig. 2) of mometasone and an antibiotic chosen based on the pre-treatment naso-endoscopic guided swab culture. These drugs are FDA approved and already being used clinically both in pill form and liquid (injectable) formulations for the treatment of infections.

Mometasone is among the most potent intranasally used steroids, in terms of its affinity with the glucocorticoid receptor(Derendorf and Meltzer, 2008). The culture-directed antibiotic is selected among several concentration-dependent agents, with minimal systemic absorption: levofloxacin, tobramycin, mupirocin, and vancomycin. The steroid/antibiotic aerosolized mixture is self-administered using a vibrating mesh nebulizer, which creates an aerosol mist by a rapidly vibrating mesh with hundreds of 4 to 8 μm holes, and allows a fast and uniform delivery of small aerosolized medication particles to the sinus walls.

In addition, endoscopic nasal toilet, with careful removal of biofilm and crusts from the sinuses, will be performed weekly by the treating rhinologist after the application of numbing spray in the nasal cavity. Following nasal toilet, topical mometasone and culture-directed antibiotic preparations are instilled inside the sinus cavities using a curved suction tip (Fig. 2). The drugs are introduced into the sinuses in a gel form (Fig. 3), which is prepared by a pharmacy, specifically for the needs of the rhinotopic protocol. Three mL of gel are instilled in each side, and distributed evenly in the maxillary sinus cavity, along the opened sphenoid and ethmoid cells, and towards the frontal recess. This drug-containing hydrophilic gel contains the non-ionic ether hydroxyethyl cellulose, which is a mucoadhesive agent. Upon its placement into the paranasal sinuses, it forms a mucoadherent film, resistant to erosion, which remains in contact with the respiratory epithelium. The prolonged attachment of the polymer matrix to the diseased mucosa, facilitates effective drug release onto the pharmacological target, and negates the mucociliary clearance of therapeutic agents(Ugwoke et al., 2005). Patients are advised to refrain from sinus rinsing or drug nebulization for the next 24 hours subsequently to gel placement.

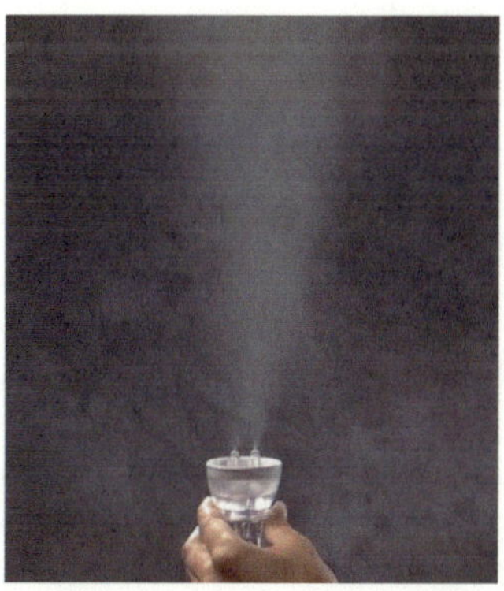

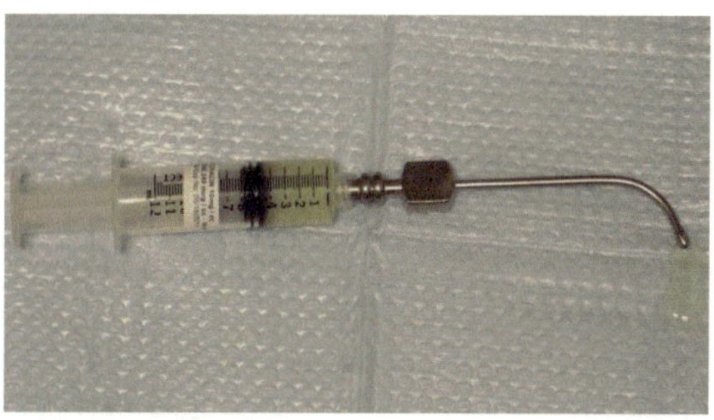

Fig. 2. The NasoNeb™ nebulizer (Left) is used for drug aerosolization in the rhinotopic protocol, and the hydroxyethyl cellulose gel (Right) is instilled through a curved suction tip.

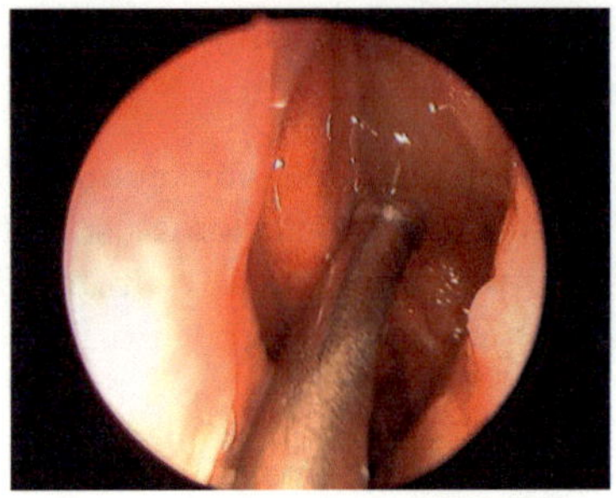

Fig. 3. The steroid & antibiotic releasing gel is introduced into the left maxillary and ethmoid cavities with a curved suction.

The duration of the protocol is six weeks, and one month later, the swab culture and the biopsy of the mucosa are repeated, to document the effect of treatment on the bacteriology, pathology, and biofilm formation.

On each patient encounter after treatment beginning (weekly debridement visits, one and two months post treatment), the clinical response to the protocol is monitored (Fig. 4). The evaluation outcome is quantified using the Lund-Kennedy (LK) symptoms score and the endoscopic appearance score(Lund and Kennedy, 1997).

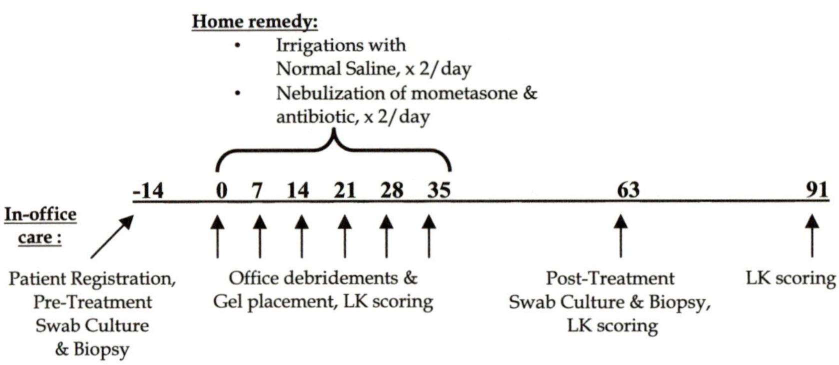

Fig. 4. Graphic of the protocol time-plan (numbers represent days).

6.2.3 Risks

The most serious possible side effects of the topical treatment protocol may include:

- Early and/or late recurrence of sinus symptoms.
- Allergic reaction to the antibiotic. If the patient has ever had any unusual or allergic reaction to any of the medications that are to be instilled, then these will be avoided, and another medication will be chosen.
- Subjects will be inconvenienced only by the need to undergo pre- and post-treatment biopsies of sinus mucosa. Bleeding, pain and infection may occur as a result of biopsies.
- Since there is minimal systemic absorption, we do not expect any immunosuppressive effect of the corticosteroids or any adrenal suppression effect. As mentioned previously, mometasone is the intranasally used steroid with the lowest systemic absorption rate (<0.1%).

6.2.4 Patient monitoring

The response to treatment is assessed by pre- and post-therapeutic evaluation of four clinicopathological parameters:

- LK symptom (Table 1) and endoscopic scores (Table 2).

Symptom	Score
Nasal blockage or congestion	0-10
Headache	0-10
Facial Pain	0-10
Hyposmia	0-10
Nasal discharge or post-nasal drip	0-10
Sneezing	0-10
Total Symptom Score	*0-60*

Table 1. Lund-Kennedy symptom scale: The patient is interviewed with regard to the severity of his symptoms over the past week, and provides a score of 0 (absent symptom) to 10 (maximum possible symptom).

Endoscopic feature	Score	
	R	L
Edema	0-2	0-2
Polyps	0-2	0-2
Discharge	0-2	0-2
Crusting	0-2	0-2
Adhesions	0-2	0-2
Total Endoscopic Score	*0-20*	

Table 2. Lund-Kennedy endoscopic appearance scale: The rhinologist assesses five endoscopic parameters on each side, providing a score of 0, 1, or 2, as follows: Edema, adhesions, and discharge: 0-absent, 1-mild, 2-severe. Polyps: 0-absent, 1-polyps only in middle meatus, 2-polyps extending beyond middle meatus. Discharge: 0-clear, 1-thin secretions, 2-thick, purulent secretions.

- Swab culture from the middle meatus.
- Histopathological diagnosis and grading of the mucosal inflammation. In detail, characteristics of chronic inflammation (epithelial necrosis, sub-mucosal edema, polypoid degeneration, lymphocyte infiltration) are identified on Hematoxylin & Eosin tissue sections.
- Biofilm quantification. A piece of the mucosa specimen is subjected to a colony forming units - assay, which provides an estimate of the biofilm's bacterial burden.

6.2.5 Rhinotopic study

In order to assess the efficacy of the rhinotopic protocol, we conducted a prospective study with the participation of 20 patients. All subjects suffered from refractory CRS, and fulfilled the inclusion criteria for receiving the rhinotopic therapy. This study tested the hypothesis that direct intra-sinus administration of antibiotics and steroids in a gel & aerosol media, in addition to frequent sinus cleansing, restores the health of the mucosa, prevents adhesion formation, reduces polyp recurrence, and eradicates sinus pathogens that are otherwise resistant to other types of treatment. We did not use a control group, because every candidate for rhinotopic therapy had been unsuccessfully treated in the past with a standard regimen of oral antibiotics, so that all controls by definition represent treatment failures.

The study population included 12 women (60%) and 8 men (40%), with age range from 13 to 76 years (mean age: 48 years). Four patients (20%) were tested positive in allergy workup (allergen-specific IgE measurement) upon enrolment, and received immunotherapy. Two patients (10%) presented with the Samter's triad of symptoms, and leukotriene inhibitors were prescribed. The most commonly cultured aerobic bacteria were Staphylococcus aureus (8 cases, 40%), and Pseudomonas aeruginosa (6 patients, 30%). Anaerobe growth was not documented. The culture-directed antibiotics that were used in the study included tobramycin in 14 cases (70%), vancomycin and levofloxacin.

Outcome measures of the sudy were the differences between pre- and post-treatment LK symptom/endoscopic scores, swab culture results, histological gravity of chronic inflammation, as well as the bacterial density of the supra-epithelial biofilm. There was a statistically significant improvement between the mean pre- and post-treatment LK symptom and endoscopic appearance scores (student's t-test, $P<0.001$). All six LK symptoms were individually improved as well. The post-treatment culture results showed no growth in 65% of the cases, normal respiratory flora in 25%, and infection by the original pathogenic organism in 10%. Comparison of histopathological findings in the pre- and post-treatment specimens, revealed a substantial reversal of almost all indices of chronic inflammation (Fig. 5). With regard to the bacterial density of biofilm, the mean number of CFUs/ml has decreased by 98.7%, one month after the completion of the rhinotopic protocol. This sharp drop clearly indicates the elimination of viable microorganisms within the biofilm matrix.

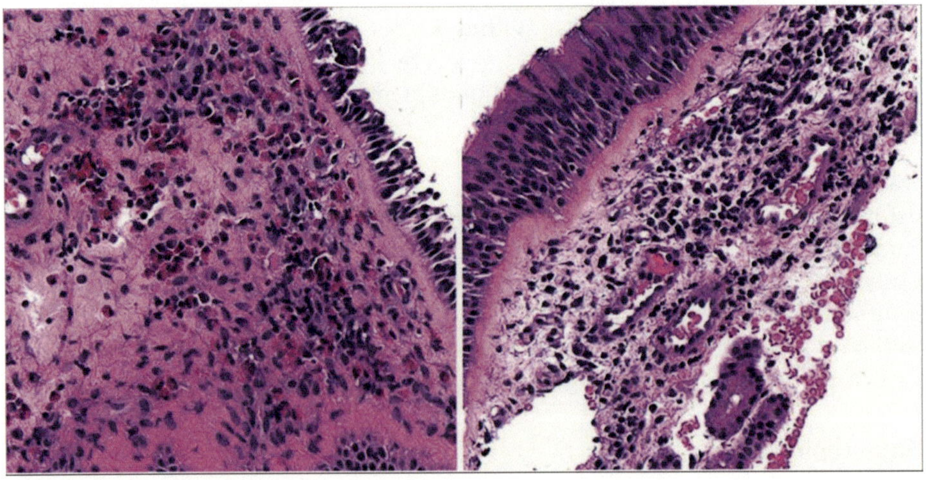

Fig. 5. Histopathological microphotographs of sinus mucosa in CRS. Left: Before the rhinotopic protocol, epithelial attenuation, disruption of epithelia layer, and marked eosinophilic inflammation are evident. Right: Post-treatment, epithelial integrity increases and inflammation resolves.

None of the patients reported any systemic or local adverse reactions. Careful endoscopy during the follow-up visits, did not reveal severe irritation, crusting, or signs of recent epistaxis.

6.2.6 The rhinotopic protocol: How it works

Refractory chronic sinusitis is a multifactorial disease, and its chronicity relies on constant debris accumulation, unremitting inflammation, and insidious infection. The optimal management needs to be multifactorial as well, and address all three components concurrently. The rhinotopic protocol is a comprehensive, strictly topical, approach to this difficult-to-treat entity. It is not applied routinely to any CRS case, but it is rather indicated for selected patients, who had previously received high-quality surgical and medical treatment, but continue to experience prolonged symptoms of moderate to severe intensity.

Mechanical cleansing by means of frequent high-pressure saline irrigations and weekly office debridements, although simple, ensures the efficacy of the pharmacological interventions. Crusts, mucopurulent secretions, and exudates, are toxic to the underlying epithelium, and perpetuate the inflammation. Meticulous removal of debris is the sine qua non of every topical therapy, in the same way it is essential for the normal healing process post-sinus surgery(Palmer and Kennedy, 2003).

The anti-inflammatory effect of the treatment is achieved by the sustained action of mometasone, one of the most potent commercially available steroids. The steroid is applied locally via a combination of two advanced delivery techniques, i.e., nebulization of small aerosolized particles, and endoscopically-guided instillation of a mucoadhesive gel. Remarkable edema reduction, and down-regulation of the eosinophilic infiltration, are among the proven consequences of systemic steroid use. Even though, this clinical improvement may not be very long-lasting. According to our data, resolution of inflammation-related symptoms, such as congestion, nasal discharge, and facial tenderness, is still documented one month after the topical protocol's completion.

Antimicrobial agents are administered simultaneously with the steroids, via the same two delivery methods. The role of infection in chronic sinusitis is unclear, and it is common belief that CRS exacerbations are pathophysiologically analogous to acute sinusitis, and should be treated as such. Typically, culture-directed systemic antibiotics may temporarily suppress the infection, but recurrence caused by the same pathogen is frequently noted(Lim et al., 2008). The sustained, highly concentrated application of antimicrobial agents directly onto the diseased membrane, according to the rhinotopic protocol, aims to eradicate the etiologic microorganism from the sinus mucosa. It is suggested that a key factor for the successful elimination of infection is overcoming the resistance of bacteria within the biofilm shelter. The antibiotic-releasing mucoadherent gel is specifically attached to this surface-organized community, and places a dense concentration of bactericidal agents at the infection site. Our findings show an impressive decline in the population of viable bacteria residing in biofilms, as assayed by Colony Forming Units cultures, following the rhinotopic therapy. This suggests that one of the mechanisms responsible for the protocol's efficacy is the disruption of biofilms. A contributing factor to the biofilm extirpation, may be the high-pressure hydrotherapy performed by the patient alternately with the antibiotic administration. Saline irrigations possibly wash out panktonik bacteria before they become fixed to sinus walls and recolonize the organic matrix(Suh et al., 2010).

7. Conclusion

Chronic rhinosinusitis is evidently a unique disease process, and far more complex than what we commonly describe as an "infection". CRS refractory to standard treatment is not an exception to the rule, but rather an increasingly occurring phenomenon. In such a chronic illness, the side-effects of systemic medications underlie the necessity of topical therapy. The latter, as this chapter has showed, is not merely restricted to placement of a drug locally, but has been developed with the help of technology into a dynamic approach, tailored to the disease's pathophysiology. Advances in endoscopy and particularly in sinus surgery, have made the paranasal cavities accessible to application of a variety of pharmacological agents.

Our proposal is an integrated topical protocol, for the restoration of the sinus mucosa homeostasis. Preliminary results are promising, and the ultimate goal of this approach is to establish a long-term effect after treatment completion, rather than transient symptom relief. Longer follow-up of patients, and modifications of the protocol guided by ongoing findings, would be the next step.

8. References

Al-Mutairi D & Kilty SJ. (2011). Bacterial biofilms and the pathophysiology of chronic rhinosinusitis. *Curr Opin Allergy Clin Immunol,* Vol. 11, No. 1, pp. 18-23, ISSN 1473-6322

Alandejani T, Marsan J, Ferris W, Slinger R, & Chan F. (2009). Effectiveness of honey on Staphylococcus aureus and Pseudomonas aeruginosa biofilms. *Otolaryngol Head Neck Surg,* Vol. 141, No. 1, pp. 114-118, ISSN 0194-5998

Antunes MB & Becker SS. (2010). The role of local steroid injection for nasal polyposis. *Curr Allergy Asthma Rep,* Vol. 10, No. 3, pp. 175-180, ISSN 1534-6315

Armengot M, Juan G, Barona R, Garin L, & Basterra J. (1994). Immotile cilia syndrome: nasal mucociliary function and nasal ciliary abnormalities. *Rhinology,* Vol. 32, No. 3, pp. 109-111, ISSN 0300-0729

Aukema AA, Mulder PG, & Fokkens WJ. (2005). Treatment of nasal polyposis and chronic rhinosinusitis with fluticasone propionate nasal drops reduces need for sinus surgery. *J Allergy Clin Immunol,* Vol. 115, No. 5, pp. 1017-1023, ISSN 0091-6749

Bendouah Z, Barbeau J, Hamad WA, & Desrosiers M. (2006). Biofilm formation by Staphylococcus aureus and Pseudomonas aeruginosa is associated with an unfavorable evolution after surgery for chronic sinusitis and nasal polyposis. *Otolaryngol Head Neck Surg,* Vol. 134, No. 6, pp. 991-996, ISSN 0194-5998

Berger WE, Ratner PH, Casale TB, Meltzer EO, & Wall GM. (2009). Safety and efficacy of olopatadine hydrochloride nasal spray 0.6% in pediatric subjects with allergic rhinitis. *Allergy Asthma Proc,* Vol. 30, No. 6, pp. 612-623, ISSN 1539-6304

Ceri H, *et al.* (1999). The Calgary Biofilm Device: new technology for rapid determination of antibiotic susceptibilities of bacterial biofilms. *J Clin Microbiol,* Vol. 37, No. 6, pp. 1771-1776, ISSN 0095-1137

Chien YW & Chang SF. (1987). Intranasal drug delivery for systemic medications. *Crit Rev Ther Drug Carrier Syst,* Vol. 4, No. 2, pp. 67-194, ISSN 0743-4863

Chiu AG, *et al.* (2008). Baby shampoo nasal irrigations for the symptomatic post-functional endoscopic sinus surgery patient. *Am J Rhinol,* Vol. 22, No. 1, pp. 34-37, ISSN 1050-6586

Daviskas E, *et al.* (1996). Inhalation of hypertonic saline aerosol enhances mucociliary clearance in asthmatic and healthy subjects. *Eur Respir J,* Vol. 9, No. 4, pp. 725-732, ISSN 0903-1936

Daviskas E & Anderson SD. (2006). Hyperosmolar agents and clearance of mucus in the diseased airway. *J Aerosol Med,* Vol. 19, No. 1, pp. 100-109, ISSN 0894-2684

Demoly P. (2008). Safety of intranasal corticosteroids in acute rhinosinusitis. *Am J Otolaryngol,* Vol. 29, No. 6, pp. 403-413, ISSN 1532-818X

Derendorf H & Meltzer EO. (2008). Molecular and clinical pharmacology of intranasal corticosteroids: clinical and therapeutic implications. *Allergy,* Vol. 63, No. 10, pp. 1292-1300, ISSN 1398-9995

Eccles R, Eriksson M, Garreffa S, & Chen SC. (2008). The nasal decongestant effect of xylometazoline in the common cold. *Am J Rhinol,* Vol. 22, No. 5, pp. 491-496, ISSN 1050-6586

Giger R, *et al.* (2003). Comparison of once- versus twice-daily use of beclomethasone dipropionate aqueous nasal spray in the treatment of allergic and non-allergic chronic rhinosinusitis. *Eur Arch Otorhinolaryngol,* Vol. 260, No. 3, pp. 135-140, ISSN 0937-4477

Gliklich RE & Metson R. (1995). The health impact of chronic sinusitis in patients seeking otolaryngologic care. *Otolaryngol Head Neck Surg,* Vol. 113, No. 1, pp. 104-109, ISSN 0194-5998

Gliklich RE & Metson R. (1998). Economic implications of chronic sinusitis. *Otolaryngol Head Neck Surg,* Vol. 118, No. 3 Pt 1, pp. 344-349, ISSN 0194-5998

Goh YH & Goode RL. (2000). Current status of topical nasal antimicrobial agents. *Laryngoscope,* Vol. 110, No. 6, pp. 875-880, ISSN 0023-852X

Gosepath J & Mann WJ. (2005). Current concepts in therapy of chronic rhinosinusitis and nasal polyposis. *ORL J Otorhinolaryngol Relat Spec,* Vol. 67, No. 3, pp. 125-136, ISSN 0301-1569

Harvey RJ & Schlosser RJ. (2009). Local drug delivery. *Otolaryngol Clin North Am,* Vol. 42, No. 5, pp. 829-845, ix, ISSN 1557-8259

Horak F & Zieglmayer UP. (2009). Azelastine nasal spray for the treatment of allergic and nonallergic rhinitis. *Expert Rev Clin Immunol,* Vol. 5, No. 6, pp. 659-669, ISSN 1744-8409

Hyo N, Takano H, & Hyo Y. (1989). Particle deposition efficiency of therapeutic aerosols in the human maxillary sinus. *Rhinology,* Vol. 27, No. 1, pp. 17-26, ISSN 0300-0729

Karagama YG, Lancaster JL, Karkanevatos A, & O'Sullivan G. (2001). Delivery of nasal drops to the middle meatus: which is the best head position? *Rhinology,* Vol. 39, No. 4, pp. 226-229, ISSN 0300-0729

Kennedy DW. (1992). Prognostic factors, outcomes and staging in ethmoid sinus surgery. *Laryngoscope,* Vol. 102, No. 12 Pt 2 Suppl 57, pp. 1-18, ISSN 0023-852X

Krouse JH. (2000). Computed tomography stage, allergy testing, and quality of life in patients with sinusitis. *Otolaryngol Head Neck Surg,* Vol. 123, No. 4, pp. 389-392, ISSN 0194-5998

Kundoor V & Dalby RN. (2010). Assessment of nasal spray deposition pattern in a silicone human nose model using a color-based method. *Pharm Res,* Vol. 27, No. 1, pp. 30-36, ISSN 1573-904X

Lavigne F, *et al.* (2002). Intrasinus administration of topical budesonide to allergic patients with chronic rhinosinusitis following surgery. *Laryngoscope,* Vol. 112, No. 5, pp. 858-864, ISSN 0023-852X

Leonard DW & Bolger WE. (1999). Topical antibiotic therapy for recalcitrant sinusitis. *Laryngoscope,* Vol. 109, No. 4, pp. 668-670, ISSN 0023-852X

Lethbridge-Cejku M, Schiller JS, & Bernadel L. (2004). Summary health statistics for U.S. adults: National Health Interview Survey, 2002. *Vital Health Stat 10,* Vol., No. 222, pp. 1-151, ISSN 0083-1972

Levine HL. (1990). Functional endoscopic sinus surgery: evaluation, surgery, and follow-up of 250 patients. *Laryngoscope,* Vol. 100, No. 1, pp. 79-84, ISSN 0023-852X

Lim M, Citardi MJ, & Leong JL. (2008). Topical antimicrobials in the management of chronic rhinosinusitis: a systematic review. *Am J Rhinol,* Vol. 22, No. 4, pp. 381-389, ISSN 1050-6586

Lund VJ & Kennedy DW. (1997). Staging for rhinosinusitis. *Otolaryngol Head Neck Surg,* Vol. 117, No. 3 Pt 2, pp. S35-40, ISSN 0194-5998

Mabry RL. (1981). Visual loss after intranasal corticosteroid injection. Incidence, causes, and prevention. *Arch Otolaryngol,* Vol. 107, No. 8, pp. 484-486, ISSN 0003-9977

Mabry RL. (1981). Evaluation of systemic absorption of intraturbinally injected triamcinolone. *Otolaryngol Head Neck Surg,* Vol. 89, No. 2, pp. 268-270, ISSN 0194-5998

Meltzer EO, *et al.* (2004). Rhinosinusitis: establishing definitions for clinical research and patient care. *J Allergy Clin Immunol,* Vol. 114, No. 6 Suppl, pp. 155-212, ISSN 0091-6749

Merkus P, Ebbens FA, Muller B, & Fokkens WJ. (2006). The 'best method' of topical nasal drug delivery: comparison of seven techniques. *Rhinology,* Vol. 44, No. 2, pp. 102-107, ISSN 0300-0729

Miller TR, Muntz HR, Gilbert ME, & Orlandi RR. (2004). Comparison of topical medication delivery systems after sinus surgery. *Laryngoscope,* Vol. 114, No. 2, pp. 201-204, ISSN 0023-852X

Moller W, Munzing W, & Canis M. (2010). Clinical potential of pulsating aerosol for sinus drug delivery. *Expert Opin Drug Deliv,* Vol. 7, No. 11, pp. 1239-1245, ISSN 1744-7593

Moss RB & King VV. (1995). Management of sinusitis in cystic fibrosis by endoscopic surgery and serial antimicrobial lavage. Reduction in recurrence requiring surgery. *Arch Otolaryngol Head Neck Surg,* Vol. 121, No. 5, pp. 566-572, ISSN 0886-4470

Nakamura K, *et al.* (1999). Uptake and release of budesonide from mucoadhesive, pH-sensitive copolymers and their application to nasal delivery. *J Control Release,* Vol. 61, No. 3, pp. 329-335, ISSN 0168-3659

Palmer JN & Kennedy DW. (2003). Medical management in functional endoscopic sinus surgery failures. *Curr Opin Otolaryngol Head Neck Surg,* Vol. 11, No. 1, pp. 6-12, ISSN 1068-9508

Papsin B & McTavish A. (2003). Saline nasal irrigation: Its role as an adjunct treatment. *Can Fam Physician,* Vol. 49, No., pp. 168-173, ISSN 0008-350X

Ponikau JU, *et al.* (1999). The diagnosis and incidence of allergic fungal sinusitis. *Mayo Clin Proc,* Vol. 74, No. 9, pp. 877-884, ISSN 0025-6196

Ranade VV. (2001). Inhalation therapy: new delivery systems. *Am J Ther,* Vol. 8, No. 5, pp. 367-381, ISSN 1075-2765

Schenkel EJ, *et al.* (2000). Absence of growth retardation in children with perennial allergic rhinitis after one year of treatment with mometasone furoate aqueous nasal spray. *Pediatrics,* Vol. 105, No. 2, pp. E22, ISSN 1098-4275

Sharp HJ, Denman D, Puumala S, & Leopold DA. (2007). Treatment of acute and chronic rhinosinusitis in the United States, 1999-2002. *Arch Otolaryngol Head Neck Surg,* Vol. 133, No. 3, pp. 260-265, ISSN 0886-4470

Shikani AH, Chahine KA, & Alqudah MA. (2010). The rhinotopic protocol for chronic refractory rhinosinusitis: how we do it. *Clin Otolaryngol,* Vol. 35, No. 4, pp. 329-332, ISSN 1749-4486

Stewart PS & Costerton JW. (2001). Antibiotic resistance of bacteria in biofilms. *Lancet,* Vol. 358, No. 9276, pp. 135-138, ISSN 0140-6736

Suh JD, Ramakrishnan V, & Palmer JN. (2010). Biofilms. *Otolaryngol Clin North Am,* Vol. 43, No. 3, pp. 521-530, viii, ISSN 1557-8259

Sykes DA, Wilson R, Chan KL, Mackay IS, & Cole PJ. (1986). Relative importance of antibiotic and improved clearance in topical treatment of chronic mucopurulent rhinosinusitis. A controlled study. *Lancet,* Vol. 2, No. 8503, pp. 359-360, ISSN 0140-6736

Tarran R, Grubb BR, Gatzy JT, Davis CW, & Boucher RC. (2001). The relative roles of passive surface forces and active ion transport in the modulation of airway surface liquid volume and composition. *J Gen Physiol,* Vol. 118, No. 2, pp. 223-236, ISSN 0022-1295

Ugwoke MI, Agu RU, Verbeke N, & Kinget R. (2005). Nasal mucoadhesive drug delivery: background, applications, trends and future perspectives. *Adv Drug Deliv Rev,* Vol. 57, No. 11, pp. 1640-1665, ISSN 0169-409X

Unno T, Hokunan K, Yanai O, & Onodera S. (1983). Deposition of sprayed particles in the nasal cavity. *Auris Nasus Larynx,* Vol. 10, No. 2, pp. 109-116, ISSN 0385-8146

Uren B, Psaltis A, & Wormald PJ. (2008). Nasal lavage with mupirocin for the treatment of surgically recalcitrant chronic rhinosinusitis. *Laryngoscope,* Vol. 118, No. 9, pp. 1677-1680, ISSN 1531-4995

Vaughan WC & Carvalho G. (2002). Use of nebulized antibiotics for acute infections in chronic sinusitis. *Otolaryngol Head Neck Surg,* Vol. 127, No. 6, pp. 558-568, ISSN 0194-5998

Wahl KJ & Otsuji A. (2003). New medical management techniques for acute exacerbations of chronic rhinosinusitis. *Curr Opin Otolaryngol Head Neck Surg,* Vol. 11, No. 1, pp. 27-32, ISSN 1068-9508

Weschta M, *et al.* (2004). Topical antifungal treatment of chronic rhinosinusitis with nasal polyps: a randomized, double-blind clinical trial. *J Allergy Clin Immunol,* Vol. 113, No. 6, pp. 1122-1128, ISSN 0091-6749

Yoo JK, Seikaly H, & Calhoun KH. (1997). Extended use of topical nasal decongestants. *Laryngoscope,* Vol. 107, No. 1, pp. 40-43, ISSN 0023-852X

Zadeh MH, Banthia V, Anand VK, & Huang C. (2002). Significance of eosinophilia in chronic rhinosinusitis. *Am J Rhinol,* Vol. 16, No. 6, pp. 313-317, ISSN 1050-6586